DATE DUE

NOV 1 6 1981		
NOV 1 9 1981		
NOV 1 9 1981		
APR 2 1 1982		
MAY 6 1982		
MAY 7 1982		
JUL 1 8 1984		
AUG 8 1984		
AUG 9 1984		
AUG 9 1984		
APR 1 1986		
	RENEWED	
APR 2 8 1986		
MAY 1 7 1988		

DEMCO 38-297

PSROs
and The Law

John D. Blum, J.D., M.Sc.
Paul M. Gertman, M.D.
Jean Rabinow, J.D.

Aspen Systems Corporation
Germantown, Maryland
1977

To the members of the Boston University PSRO Project

Table of Contents

Preface

ON THE INEVITABILITY OF CHANGE

This book discusses the law governing peer review. Special attention is paid to Professional Standards Review Organizations (PSROs) because most of the legal action (not to mention most of the debate) in the peer review field has been generated by the PSRO program, and will probably continue to be unless the PSRO program is discontinued.

Because the PSRO program has generated significant legal activity, the law itself is in flux. Therefore, those who read this book in search of the one right way to run a peer review program (or the one best way to attack it in court) are bound to be disappointed. In fact, even if the PSRO law had not been enacted, if PSRO regulations were not being periodically issued, and if no one were taking the federal government to court to force them to abolish or amend the PSRO law, the law's normal unpredictability would still prevent any plan of action or line of attack from being characterized as completely safe.

What is this "normal unpredictability"? While many laymen are willing to accept the idea that two different juries can take one set of laws and similar facts and nevertheless come up with two diametrically opposed decisions, fewer realize that the law itself is inherently less than precise. While it is probably fair to say that a large percentage (perhaps the majority) of students entering law school, nonprofessionals all, have come there partly to find in the legal system a solidity, a bedrock on which to build a structure of morality and justice in a world subject to moral ambiguity and change, one of the first things they learn—and it is one of the hardest lessons—is that the law is not solid bedrock; often it most closely resembles quicksand.

To the lawyers who may read this book, this revelation is nothing new. To the other readers, a warning is perhaps in order: when you deal with the law, particularly in a developing field like modern medical law, you are entering a swamp after dark. Any map you may be fortunate enough to have been given—such as this book—was printed a day, a week, or a year ago, and could well have been created by a guide whose familiarity with your particular swamp, no matter how great his experience with other and perhaps closely similar swamps, is only slightly greater than your own. The law can change faster than books can be published, and the facts can change faster than the law.

Then can a guidebook be useful at all? Absolutely. One reason is that although there have been very few statutes enacted, regulations promulgated, or cases litigated about peer review or PSRO, there have been some; and an impartial (in the sense of nonpartisan or nonparticipant) discussion of these statutes, regulations, and cases can be useful. A second reason is that even though there is little precedent in the field of PSRO, peer review, and the law, sufficient parallels exist in other legal areas so that interested lawyers will be able to fashion arguments based on analogies wherever legal precedent is lacking. A consideration of some of those parallels can help lawyer and physician alike: the lawyer, to fashion arguments; the physician, to see what the arguments are likely to be.

We make no promises that this book will be entirely current, either about the state of the law or about the facts (we sincerely hope, for example, that HEW will have issued several new sets of PSRO regulations by the time this is published). We have become increasingly aware of the need to warn that nothing contained in this book is to be taken as legal advice. It is certainly not intended to be legal advice. At best, this book can be, to return to the metaphor, a map as current as we can make it, and which will be most useful to physician-lawyer teams as they set out together into the swamp of peer review law. For the actual organizing and operation of peer review programs (inside the PSRO program or out), physicians will be needed; for the interpreting of various statutes and the litigating of court cases, lawyers. If this book can be useful to each group in performing their jobs and in their efforts to communicate to each other what has to be done, it will have served its purpose.

In trying to make this book useful to a broad spectrum of those involved in PSRO and/or other peer review programs, we have had to strike a balance between discussion of peer review methodologies and discussion of legal technicalities. In general, the first and third chapters contain the bulk of the book's material on peer review programs and methodologies, and on the "nonlegal" concerns that shape those programs and will ultimately shape the law. Chapters two and four through eight discuss "the law" as it exists and as it will ultimately shape medical peer review programs; the legal issues of constitutionality, confidentiality, agency, malpractice, and corporate liability are dealt with in detail. We have tried to keep the vocabulary of both kinds of chapters from becoming overly technical, and have tried to explain the technical terms needed to avoid ambiguity or prolixity. The main exception to this rule of semitechnicality is that we have assumed throughout that the readers —you—will understand how the American legal system works, at least in a general way. For those who are neither lawyers nor physicians with legal experience, we recommend highly the reading of Appendix A. Much of what follows will be gibberish to those who do not understand the distinction between federal and state law; between legislative (statute), executive (regulation), and judicial (case or "common-law" law); and between state prosecution and private lawsuit.

Our other warning is that certain subjects will appear repeatedly in different chapters and sections. We regret that this cannot be helped. Certain sections of the PSRO statute, for example, are relevant to questions of both confidentiality and corporate liability. Some of the material on agency is indispensible to any discussion of constitutionality. We hope that our text will make these different aspects entirely clear.

John D. Blum, J.D., M.Sc.
Jean Rabinow, J.D.
Boston, Massachusetts
May 1977

AUTHORS' NOTE

With the creation of the Health Care Financing Administration, the Bureau of Quality Assurance is to become the Health Standards and Quality Bureau in the new agency. Because the change to the Health Standards and Quality Bureau is so recent this text still refers to the PSRO federal administrative agency as BQA. This organizational development does not substantially affect the content of this book.

* * *

Concerning the discussion in Chapter 2, final reimbursement policies for hospital-based review were issued by BQA in Transmittal 46. Payment for PSRO review is to be made through Medicare and Medicaid trust funds. Under Transmittal 46 each delegated hospital is required to develop an estimated unit cost per admission. Provisions are also included to allow for retroactive payment to February 1, 1976.

June 1977

Chapter 1

The Development of Peer Review

This chapter discusses some of the major developments that have shaped medical peer review procedures and programs. The presentation is largely historical, detailing the movement from voluntary to mandatory peer review efforts. Background information is included on utilization review and medical audit, the two basic methods of conducting medical peer review.

Medical peer review has historically moved from voluntary efforts in upgrading the quality of medical care to government-mandated medical peer review programs, most recently the PSRO program. Three primary developments have occurred: accreditation of facilities; cost review mechanisms; and medical audit. For our purposes, the term "medical audit" will be used to describe a method of retrospective review referred to in the PSRO program as "medical care evaluation." Technically speaking, medical audit could be described as one type of medical care evaluation.

EARLY DEVELOPMENTS

Formal peer review dates back to the early twentieth century, when medicine was becoming an increasingly scientific discipline and professional conscience was aroused by two studies: the Flexner Report on the inadequacy of medical education; and a study of hospital facilities by the American College of Surgeons, which found that most institutions surveyed were unable to meet any reasonable standard of quality.[1] At the same time, a type of medical audit emerged in the work of Dr. Ernest Codman, who devised techniques for the evaluation of medical care and the correction of treatment errors.[2]

1

For the next thirty years, however, most of the activity in medical quality control focused on facilities and operational standards, as can be seen by the enactment of hospital licensing statutes. Eventually, these efforts culminated in the creation of the Joint Commission on Accreditation of Hospitals (JCAH).[3] Activities to upgrade medical practice standards were largely voluntary efforts by medical societies or hospital staff committees (such as tissue review committees). In the 1950s, beginning with the work of Dr. Paul Lembcke, significant research began in measuring the quality of medical care.[4] Lembcke conducted a pilot program in Rochester, New York, which collected clinical information to improve the equality of medical care in participating hospitals.[5]

Another experimental medical audit program, undertaken in Southwestern Michigan, was the Professional Activities Study (PAS) sponsored by the American College of Surgeons.[6] The Michigan study developed a system in which data collected from patients' medical records made up uniform patient abstracts to aid medical audit committees in selecting cases and types of patient care for study.[7] "As a follow-up to the work of PAS the Commission on Professional and Hospital Activities (CPHA) was founded in 1955. Its intent was to gather clinical information about the practices in hospitals into one centralized research file which would be available on a national basis. CPHA joined with the American College of Surgeons on related research activities which led to the establishment of the Medical Audit Program (MAP)."[8]

The early 1960s saw the creation of a number of successful quality review programs, including the Hospital and Medical Economics Study in Michigan; the Hospital Utilization Program in Western Pennsylvania; and the Pilot Study of Hospital Use in Nassau County, New York.[9] The Michigan Hospital and Medical Economics Study found in its evaluation of hospital utilization that appropriateness of admission, length of stay, and diagnostic procedures all had pertinence in measuring the quality of medical care as well as the effectiveness of hospital use.[10]

One of the methods encouraged by federal and private insurers to control expenditures was utilization review (UR). Early efforts in organized UR activities can be traced to Western Pennsylvania, where guidelines were developed by the Allegheny County Medical Society, for Blue Cross, to establish UR committees in the 1950s. This was the first major review effort that focused on both the cost and the quality of care. From these efforts in Pennsylvania, the Hospital Utilization Project (HUP) was formed to provide data service support and technical consulting for UR activities in Western Pennsylvania (much like the PAS system).[11]

Utilization review first became mandatory in 1965 with passage of the Medicare law. Government involvement with peer review since 1965 gives evidence of two definite trends: First, the government's desire to delegate the review task to physician committees; and second, the government's inability to settle on an acceptable review methodology. Government review delegation can be attributed to both a lack of manpower and a wish to temper governmental control over review to make it more acceptable to the medical profession.

The Medicare Law[12] made hospital-based utilization review committees a requirement for participation in Medicare reimbursement. Title XVIII of the Social Security Act required that participating hospitals and extended care facilities establish a plan for utilization review and that a standing UR committee be maintained:

1. for the review, on a sample or other basis, of admissions to the institution, the duration of stays therein, and the professional services (including drugs and biologicals) furnished (A) in respect to medical needs of the service; and (B) the purpose of promoting the most efficient use of available health facilities and services;

2. for such review to be made by either: (A) a staff committee of the institution composed of two or more physicians, with or without participation of other professional personnel; or (B) a group outside the institution which is similarly composed and (i) which is established by the local medical society and some or all of the hospitals and extended care facilities in the locality, or (ii) if (and for as long as) there has not been established such a group which serves such institution, which is established in such other manner as may be approved by the Secretary;

3. for such review, in each case of inpatient hospital services or extended care services furnished to such an individual during a continuous period of extended duration, as of such days of such period (which may differ for different classes of cases) as may be specified in regulations, with such review to be made as promptly as possible, after each day so specified, and in no event later than one week following such day; and

4. for prompt notification to the institution, the individual, and his attending physician of any finding (made after opportunity for consultation to such attending physician) by the physician members of such committee or group that any further stay in the institution is not medically necessary.

The review committee must be composed as provided in clause (B) of paragraph (2) rather than as provided in clause (A) of such paragraph in the case of any hospital or extended care facility where, because of the small size of the institution, of (in the case of an extended care facility) because of lack of an organized medical staff, or for such other reason or reasons as may be included in regulations, it is impracticable for the institution to have a properly functioning staff committee for the purposes of this subsection.

Utilization review committees were the major check against overuse of services included in the statute. UR, when combined with specific conditions of participation for providers and with physician certification, was geared toward insuring that medical services would only be provided where actually needed. As one student of Blue Cross observed, "The institutional utilization review committee was to make the final judgment on the medical necessity of care provided to Medicare beneficiaries. The legislative history indicates that Congress was fully aware that, whatever dangers might be involved in placing the final determination of medical necessity in the hands of the professional committee within the provider institution, that was the way it was to be."[13]

While Utilization Review under Title XVIII (and later XIX) was designed to be a useful tool to gain medical information and to act as a means of continuing physician education, its main thrust was cost control. Sample retrospective review was to be adopted as an effective method to identify abuses in institutional admissions, services, and patterns of care, without placing undue pressure on providers or practitioners. Extended stay review, on the other hand, was designed to prevent lengthy hospital stays that represented the greatest cost strain on the system. Thus the federal government attempted to build into a costly system a method to economize in the area of greatest abuse, which was felt to be extended stay. Concentration in this area required only minimal interference with medical practice, as indicated in the preamble of the Medicare statute.

The early experience with utilization review under Medicare proved in general to be a failure. A Senate committee found that "UR Committees have not made the reviews required by their own plans, have not consulted with attending physicians on a timely basis, and have not informed patients or institutions of their decisions."[14] A lack of physician commitment to and understanding of the Title XVII UR process, together with the failure of the Social Security Administration and fiscal intermediaries to educate physicians adequately about the program, rendered review efforts highly ineffective.[15]

In the private sector, peer review developed under the auspices of the Joint Commission on Accreditation of Hospitals (JCAH), the AMA, and other organized medical groups, largely in response to government control. Medical peer review was approached by organized medicine as an educational tool designed to upgrade the quality of care. Its use as a mandatory process, with potential punishments, was rejected.

After 1965, the JCAH took on the function of hospital certification. Under the then-new Medicare law, a JCAH-accredited facility with an acceptable utilization review plan was eligible to receive payment under Title XVIII. The JCAH, by virtue of the Medicare law, had in effect become a quasi-public licensing authority. With its expanded role, the Commission found itself being criticized for the vagueness of its guidelines by federal officials, hospital groups, and consumers, and was forced to implement more stringent standards.[16]

PEER REVIEW METHODOLOGIES

At this point it should be helpful to review the two basic methodologies that have been and still are employed in public and private sector review programs: Utilization review and medical audit.

Utilization review is designed to aid in making the medical treatment process cost-effective, mainly through analyzing institutional length-of-stay and hospital bed utilization. *Medical audit* primarily examines the quality of care and the types of services provided in the institution. Professional evaluation of physician services can focus on any type of treatment setting, from office visits to clinics, nursing homes, and acute-care hospitals.

The following descriptions of utilization review and medical audit are based on general models. There are numerous variations for both UR and medical audit systems, but overall, principles basic to these review methodologies can be identified.

Utilization Review Under Current Law

The function of a hospital utilization review committee is "to minimize the cost of patient care by monitoring the use of the hospital and its resources, primarily so that excess usage (and cost) is prevented," according to the American Hospital Association.[17] If review is to be cost-effective, inappropriate admissions, unnecessary hospital stay, and overutilization of hospital ancillary services must all be considered. Utilization review can take place at any of three times in relation to the service provided: it can be *prospective, concurrent,* or *retrospective.*

Prospective review involves preadmission certification for elective hospital admissions. The purpose of preadmission certification is to insure that the hospital is the proper setting for providing the treatment a patient requires. This is accomplished in two ways: (1) By reviewing admissions against implicit or explicit admission criteria for the most common diseases; (2) by prospective authorization for a length-of-stay based on empiric, average regional or national experience for that specific disease.[18]

Preadmission certification (as well as concurrent review) analyzes each hospital admission on the basis of what the utilization review committee or the PSRO feels are justifiable reasons. A length-of-stay range is assigned to each admission based upon experience within the hospital or data derived from the area.[19]

Concurrent review is ordinarily used to monitor the appropriateness of the utilization of hospital beds and/or other facilities, and is applied to any admission, whether emergency or elective, within a certain number of hours after the patient has entered the institution.[20] The number and types of cases reviewed will depend on the specific review program. Although concurrent review can be limited to "problem" cases, federal regulations appear to require more extensive (total) review.[21] In concurrent review, a specific time period, based upon the admitting diagnostic category, is assigned to the patient's hospital stay. Length-of-stay determinations were originally based upon an arbitrarily fixed period, but now a certified length-of-stay for a given diagnosis usually represents an average (often the 50th percentile) stay, based on regional or national statistics. When the initial length-of-stay period is about to expire, if a request for additional days is made, an extension may be granted. Prior to an extension's approval, the case will be re-reviewed (continued-stay review) to determine whether or not there is medical necessity for continued hospitalization.[22]

The following is a typical model based on procedures used in a concurrent review setting. It is not, however, meant to represent all utilization review programs.

A physician, upon requesting admission of his patient, supplies the medical information necessary to complete an admission certification request form.

Within a specified time after the patient is admitted to the hospital, the review coordinator (patient care coordinator, program coordinator, nurse reviewer) examines the patient's medi-

cal record to determine if the admission is "medically necessary." The determination of medical necessity will be made on
the basis of criteria established by the utilization review committee for the admitting diagnosis in question. If the coordinator is satisfied that the patient meets the UR criteria, the admission is certified and an initial length-of-stay is assigned on
the basis of the patient's age, diagnosis, and regional norms. If
the review coordinator finds that the admission criteria are not
fulfilled, or is uncertain whether or not the patient stay should
be certified, the case is referred to a physician advisor.

The physician advisor, once a case is referred to him, has
three options: (1) To certify the admission and assign a three-
day initial length-of-stay, (2) to certify the admission and assign a three-day initial length-of-stay if the admitting diagnosis
is preliminary or unclear, (3) to consult with the attending physician to allow that individual the opportunity to present his
views.

If a consensus between the admitting physician and the physician advisor cannot be reached, a peer review committee will
resolve the issue. The peer review committee, which may in
fact be composed of one physician, has the final say in determining medical necessity. If the committee concludes that the
admission is medically indicated, the physician advisor and the
coordinator will be told to certify the admission and assign an
initial length-of-stay. If the peer review committee determines
that hospitalization is not required, written notices so stating
are sent to the attending physician, patient (or next of kin),
hospital administration, and where appropriate, the third-
party payer.

If the patient's admission has been certified and a length-of-
stay assigned, the review coordinator will be responsible for assessing the patient's progress. Within a set period of time prior
to the expiration of the assigned length-of-stay (often 2 days
before) the coordinator will review the patient's record, using
criteria established for the diagnosis in question. If additional
hospitalization is indicated, the record is recertified for an extended number of hospital days on the basis of local standards.
If the review coordinator is unable to approve the extended
stay or has some question about it, the case is referred back to
the physician advisor. The physician advisor, if he fails to find
medical necessity, will consult with the attending physician; if
no agreement can be reached, the case will be referred to the

peer review committee. In the event the committee certifies the admission, an extended length-of-stay will be assigned and the recertification process will be repeated.

The "discharge planning" phase of concurrent review begins on a set date prior to the patient's planned discharge date, usually 1–2 days. At this time the coordinator reviews the record to determine whether sufficient evidence is present for discharge planning to commence. If the information in the record is adequate, the coordinator or other responsible hospital employee determines the available resources for post-discharge care and the mechanisms of transfer to other levels of care. If questions arise in the discharge planning process, the physician advisor should be consulted, and he may in turn wish to discuss the matter with the attending physician and the patient's family prior to making recommendations.[23]

Utilization review programs also frequently use the technique of *retrospective review,* which begins after a patient has been discharged. Retrospective UR is usually used to determine medical necessity and appropriateness of care by examining the collected patient data. The patient's record, selected on the basis of criteria and standards set by the UR Committee, is "pulled" and certain data abstracted. The collected data are assessed for evidence of the need for treatment, length-of-stay, type of services, level of medical practice, etc. On the basis of data analysis, the UR Committee may draft certain reports (e.g., admission and discharge analysis, length-of-stay comparison, surgical procedure index) that are helpful in illustrating institutional care.

Medical Audit

Medical audit is a general term for a method of peer review to assess the quality of care through a retrospective examination of certain key elements (critical criteria) in given diagnostic categories. Audits are conducted by groups of physicians who examine either the "process" (methods) or "outcomes" (results) of treatment, with an emphasis on uncovering overall patterns of patient care. Process medical audit examines whether specified procedures thought necessary for the patient are in fact being done. Outcome audit, on the other hand, assesses medical care by looking at the condition of patients during and after treatment and comparing the findings with hospital, regional, or national standards.

While the methods used in medical audits vary, audit can be basically understood as a series of steps: selection of the study topic, selection of a time frame, development of criteria, chart review, committee analysis, and implementation of a corrective action plan.[24]

In selecting a topic to be studied, the audit committee focuses on discharge diagnoses that are most frequently encountered or that present the most severe treatment problems. Randomly selecting discharge diagnoses for audit subject matter is not an accurate way of pinpointing problem areas; a method of topic selection more likely to reveal areas in which care can be improved is to obtain a medical staff or audit committee consensus on what diagnostic areas present the most problems. Topic selection should involve consideration of the severity of the illness, the extent to which adequate care can prevent injury to the patient, and an analysis of whether an audit can cause positive change. Topic selection may dictate the time period within which the audit will be conducted and the number of charts that must be included, although in some instances these can be left to committee discretion.

The next major stage in audit is the development by the audit committee of appropriate criteria for evaluation. Criteria having been broken down into four major types: "(a) indications for admissions; (b) hospital services recommended for optimal care; (c) range of length of stay and indications for discharge and; (d) complications for additional diagnoses." A delineation of criteria can also be broken down into therapeutic process criteria and outcome-at-discharge criteria. "Process" criteria can be developed by a method like the following; first, the indications for admissions are discussed and agreed upon, considering diagnosis and possible care. Some, but not all, admissions are clearly necessary by the time a diagnosis is suspected or, in surgical cases, by the time an operation is planned. Some admissions are discretionary; some may be contraindicated. Criteria must at least distinguish between the groups and may distinguish between "good" and "bad" discretionary decisions.

Second, the hospital services recommended for optimum care are discussed and agreed upon—the diagnostic procedure and then the optimum therapeutic procedures themselves. Significant "negative" values are also recorded here, such as the avoidance of morphine in bronchial asthma, or the avoidance of anticoagulants in peptic ulcer and other bleeding states.

Third, the optimum length of stay, or range of stay, is recorded. It may be easier to choose a fairly narrow range of stay rather than a single date because of conflicting experience of panel members, different therapeutic approaches, and, most important, the unknown in the equation—the patient himself.

Finally, complications or additional diagnoses requiring additional care and days of stay are considered, and recorded in as much detail as seems appropriate. The criteria are ready for use.

In the development of criteria, a committee generally attempts to reach some consensus as to what criteria should be adopted. Failure to reach a consensus may indicate that the criterion involved should not be used. Some audit committees do not develop their own criteria, but may borrow all or part of already-existing sets such as the diagnostic criteria established by the AMA or length of stay guidelines created by PAS.

Once criteria have been agreed upon, the actual review begins, following a three-stage process: screening, data review, and medical evaluation. A record analyst (e.g., medical record librarian, nurse) screens patients' charts in the diagnostic category being studied. The initial screener compares information in the patients' charts with the committee's criteria; results of the screening process are recorded on special worksheets. Generally, the completed worksheets contain information sufficient to enable the committee to act. In some instances, where the screening isolates problems, the committee may need one or more medical records in addition to the worksheets in order to perform adequate review.

It is the audit committee's task to evaluate whether or not the variations from the criteria were clinically justified. Deficiencies are documented and analyzed to determine to what or whom they can be attributed, i.e., the institution, the individual physician, the nursing staff, etc. The data analyzed by the committee for a given audit is compiled by committee aides (or by machine) according to key medical variables.

After the audit, the committee reports its findings, the types of evaluations made, and the criteria used. The report should be sent to the audit committee's parent organization (PSRO, hospital, or whatever) as well as to the reviewed physicians, nurses, etc.

The medical audit must also result in recommendations for corrective action whenever deficiencies are uncovered. Corrective action can take the form of suggested or required continuing education, individual counseling, reduction in staff privileges, alteration of institutional procedures, etc., depending upon the type of deficiency uncovered. Corrective action recommendations are passed to the appropriate person in the institution (whoever has the authority either to implement the recommendation or to initiate further studies). Serious deficiencies in institutional care may result in the implementation of concurrent monitoring for a specific problem area, to continue until a positive change has occurred.[25]

Medical audit could be expanded to areas other than quality review, becoming a tool to evaluate physician behavior in determining hospital privileges or to uncover administrative problems. Many methodologies for medical audit are inadequate and have been subject to widespread criticism, although few alternative systems have been developed. Besides methodology weakness, a fundamental problem is the lack of understanding of medical audit in general by health professionals.

CURRENT DEVELOPMENTS

Federal Programs

The 1967 Social Security Amendments (PL 90-248) required state Medicaid agencies to establish utilization review procedures for care and services provided under Title XIX medical assistance plans. The types of medical review conducted by states under the auspices of Title XIX vary. In some states, review procedures paralleled the Medicare system, but in other states UR included preadmission certification as a cost-control method.

One outgrowth of early UR shortcomings was the shifting of authority to the fiscal intermediaries, usually Blue Cross. As the author of *Blue Cross: What Went Wrong* pointed out: "Rather than undertaking the difficult task of monitoring hospitals and physicians with respect to Utilization Review and physicians with respect to Utilization Review and physician certification requirements, in 1967 HEW authorized Blue Cross to institute retroactive review of the medical necessity of care provided in specific cases and to deny payment where care was not medically necessary."[26] While statutory power to determine medical necessity still rested with the hospitals' UR committees, in effect the fiscal intermediary had the final power of denial, and the UR committee decision was only one factor to be considered.[27]

HEW did not issue review guidelines to the various intermediaries, but allowed each plan to develop independent methods. "Within plans, claims review ranges from auditing hospital bills to more sophisticated review of appropriateness of admissions, appropriateness of service, length of stay, deficiency in scheduling and so forth. The majority of U.S. Blue Cross Plans review all claims for appropriateness of admissions, and many review them for length of stay, appropriateness of service to specific diagnoses."[28] Some of the plans place emphasis on assisting provider UR committees; others stress physician recertification programs, and some even have medical society review committees. The emphasis of the fiscal intermediaries' reviews is clearly on cost savings. The Blue Cross study noted, "In March 1970 HEW conducted a Contract Performance Review of the New York Blue Cross Plan and recommended that the Plan consider information and educational aspects of its utilization review program as secondary and proceed to use the program to deny and reduce bills."[29]

Problems continued in the Title XVIII (and XIX) programs under fiscal intermediary review. Discrepancies in determining reasonable charges and in determining needed services, coupled with physician resentment that medical determinations were being challenged by insurance companies, proved troublesome. The Senate Finance Committee, in its 1972 report, concluded that "in light of shortcomings . . . the critically important utilization review process must be restructured and made more effective through substantially increased professional participation. The committee believes that the review process should be based upon the premise that only physicians, in general, are qualified to judge whether services ordered by other physicians are necessary."[30]

Criticism of the UR program led to changes in the UR process. Significant expansion of Medicaid review occurred with the passage of the 1972 Social Security Amendments (P.L. 92-603). Under the 1972 amendments, UR committees are required to conduct concurrent review of Title XIX hospital admission. The 1972 amendments attempted to replace fiscal intermediary determinations by returning to use of professional review committees, which would allow for the adoption of a single review program in a given state.[31] HEW's regulations under the 1972 amendments also mandated significant changes in the utilization review process. Under regulations pursuant to §237 of the law, UR committees are required to engage in concurrent review of the necessity for hospital admissions for all Title XVIII and XIX patients.[32] Extended stay review is also required for covered hospital and long-term care patients. Physician review committees are required to establish norms, standards, and criteria to use in evaluating admissions and continued stay. Nonphysicians are responsible for the initial screening of cases to be reviewed. These changes were designed to make the UR process closely resemble the most significant features contained in §249F of PL 92-603, which established the Professional Standards Review Organization program.

The new utilization review regulations, scheduled to be implemented on February 1, 1975, were challenged by a suit brought against HEW by the American Medical Association.[33] The AMA claimed that the UR regulations were an illegal interference in physicians' practice of medicine; the requirement that concurrent review be conducted within 24 hours after hospital admission was judged by the AMA and later the court to interfere with the physicians' practice and constituted a denial of treatment to the patient.[34] The AMA succeeded in enjoining the enforcement of HEW's first UR regulations. As a result, a modified set of review requirements, prepared by HEW in consultation with the AMA, appeared in March of 1976.

The issuance of the new UR regulations sparked further controversy, but a compromise resulted in greater flexibility in admission review, although the law's emphasis clearly remains cost containment. Another and more significant outgrowth of the 1972 amendments was the creation of the Professional Standards Review Organizations (PSRO), designed to take over all federal medical review activities.[35]

The UR regulations published in the November 29, 1974, *Federal Register* were said to have been designed to act as a building block for PSRO activities. "The UR regulations were designed to facilitate full transition from these activities to the PSRO review system. The Utilization Review system required by the regulations was made nearly identical to the PSRO system for this purpose."[36] The rationale for the proposed changeover to PSRO review is the avoidance of costly duplicative efforts. In these cases where there has been a waiver[37] in favor of state Medicaid agency review for both Title XIX and XVIII patients, the PSRO will also supplant state agency utilization review. The state is supposed to retain the authority to monitor the PSRO on a sample basis to determine whether the PSRO's review process corresponds to HEW regulations.[38]

Nonfederal and Joint Programs

In the private sector, both cost and quality peer review are conducted by foundations for medical care (FMCs). Foundations vary considerably in organization and function, but basically an FMC is a locally-run physician corporation whose services include either claims review or some type of prepaid health care services or a combination of both.[39] Peer review activities have been pioneered by a number of foundations, but foundation review efforts became significant only after the inception of utilization review in the 1960s.

A contribution made by the FMCs to peer review methodologies has been the development of inhospital patient certification programs. The best known of these programs, The Certified Hospital Admission Program (CHAP) was started by the Sacramento FMC in the late 1960s. Initially an attempt to check the rapidly increasing use of foundation health care services, it has now taken on a quality-of-care review component.[40] The CHAP program has been adopted, with some slight variations, by other foundations. Similar certification mechanisms are now used in New Mexico (HAPP), Utah (OSCHUR), and Illinois (HASP), among others. A number of foundations have contracted with states to perform the states' Medicaid patient review.[41]

Basically, in foundation certification programs, the attending physician provides necessary medical information so that admission certification can be granted by the foundation coordinator on the basis of established guidelines. Requests that cannot be approved are referred to a review physician for decision. Once the admission is approved, an initial length of stay is assigned to the patient on the basis of the approved admitting diagnosis. Extended hospital stays are granted if there is a request by the attending physician and medical documentation. Emergency admissions are initially certified for a set number of hours and later reviewed to determine if the admission was an emergency and to assign a length of stay. The duties and authority of the review coordinator vary in the different foundation programs, but it is clear that the coordinator is the key figure in the initial stages of the review process.

A detailed discussion of the methodology of the various inhospital certification programs is beyond the scope of this text. The fact must be recognized that these foundation certification programs have resulted in some significant savings.[42] For purposes of this discussion, the importance of programs such as CHAP or HASP is that they developed an efficient monitoring technique that serves as the basis for the PSRO review methodology.

The Experimental Medical Care Review Organizations (EMCROs), set up in 1970 by the National Center for Health Services Research (NCHSR, now NCHSR&D) as pilot projects funded by grants, were the direct precursors of the PSROs. The purpose of the EMCRO project was to develop working models that would act as testing grounds on a local level for different types of medical peer review plans.[43] Twelve EMCRO grants were ultimately awarded, the majority sponsored by foundation groups. These for the most part had some experience in doing review, and had established relationships with the necessary components fiscal intermediaries, state agencies, hospitals of the health system in their area. Each EMCRO contracted with the third parties in its area (for example, Blue Cross/Blue Shield, Title XIX) to review their patient populations. The majority of EMCROs did not limit their review activities to participating physicians but reviewed cases of all area physicians.[44]

EMCROs were supposed to measure the quality and appropriateness of care, but just how well they did is open to question. The EMCRO effort was usurped by the creation of the PSRO program, and thus its short life span prevented adequate analysis of whether quality was affected by EMCRO review. There is some evidence that EMCROs did result in decreased expenditures, but evaluation of their financial impact is not complete.[45]

Government-mandated peer review has acted to stimulate further development in this area in the private sector. The AMA, JCAH, AHA, etc., have all been significantly involved in establishing peer review programs. In fact, a degree of competition exists between private groups for hospital participation in their respective review systems. While there is tension between organized medicine and government peer review organizations, HEW has relied on private groups to develop criteria and review methodologies, as evidenced by significant funding support for such activities. The government-mandated peer review programs, being developmental, allow for flexibility in types of approaches, thus leaving a significant role for the private sector in pioneering alternative methodologies. Organized medical groups have not been squeezed out of peer review efforts, but have been able to influence government efforts as a result of their strong lobbying power. Medical organizations,with the exception of certain state medical societies, have gone above the PSRO bureaucracy to the Secretary of HEW, to the Congress, and to the courts when they desired specific policy changes, rather than encouraging local resistance.

CONCLUSION

Both the PSRO and federal UR programs place faith, time, and money in medical audit, which at present is still largely developmental and in which no methodology has yet proven to be clearly superior. From a legal standpoint, medical audit as a system that reviews thousands of medical records poses some threat to both physician and patient privacy, and it is not clear that either Title XI (PSRO) or Titles XVIII and XIX (Medicare and Medicaid) of the Social Security Act give

HEW the right to require that medical audits be part of anyone's review program, or even to fund medical audit review. However, medical audit in any of its forms promises to be a more effective quality-control method than does utilization review, and might be as effective as UR in controlling costs; current federal efforts are placing significant emphasis upon audit procedures.

NOTES

1. Paul Lembcke, "Evolution of the Medical Audit," *JAMA* 199 (1967): 111.

2. Id. at 112.

3. Carl Schlicke, "American Surgery's Noblest Experiment," *Arch. Surg.* 106 (1973): 379.

4. Lembcke, "Evolution of the Medical Audit," p. 111.

5. Kuehn, "The Commission on Professional and Hospital Activities," *Bulletin of the American College of Surgeons* 58, no. 10 (1973): 7.

6. Id.

7. Id.

8. CPHA, *PAS: Professional Activities Study—Map: Medical Audit Program* (Ann Arbor: CPHA, 1973).

9. Arthur D. Little, *An Evaluation of the Effectiveness of Utilization Review Activities in Hospitals and Extended Care Facilities* (Cambridge: Arthur D. Little, 1971).

10. B. Payne, "Medical Care Appraisal," *JAMA* 201, no. 7 (1967): 128.

11. Arthur D. Little, *An Evaluation.*

12. Medicare Law, Title XVIII, Social Security Act.

13. S. Law, *Blue Cross: What Went Wrong* (New Haven: Yale University Press, 1974).

14. U.S. Senate Finance Committee, Subcommittee on Health, *Implementation of PSRO Legislation,* Part 2 of 2 Parts, 93rd Congress (1974): 520.

15. Id.

16. A. Bryant, G. Updegraff, *Regulation of Institutional Quality* (Denver: Policy Center Inc., 1975).

17. American Hospital Association. *Quality Assurance Program* (Chicago: American Hospital Association, 1971), Sec. 12, p. 38.

18. P. Bonner, B. Decker, *PSRO: Organization for Regional Peer Review* (Cambridge: Ballinger, 1973), p. 36.

19. Id.

20. Flasher; Reed; and White, "The Hospital Admission & Surveillance Program in Illinois," *JAMA* 221, no. 10 (1972): 1153.

21. Id.

22. AHA, Quality Assurance Program, p. 55.

23. Id. at Chapter 6.

24. C.E. Lewis, "The State of the Art of Quality Assessment 1973," *Medical Care* 12, no. 10 (1974): 803. See also, R.H. Brook, "Quality Assurance—the State of the Art," *Hospital Medical Staff* (March 1974): 18.

25. Id.

26. S. Law, p. 121.

27. Id. at 122.

28. James Ensign, "Third Party Review Programs from the Blue Cross Vantage Point," *JAMA* 196, no. 11 (1966): 1006.

29. S. Law, p. 126.

30. U.S. Senate Finance Committee Report, p. 519.

31. P.L. 92-603, §1861(K).

32. Id.

33. American Medical Association v. Weinberger, 522 F. 2d 921 (1975).

34. Id.

35. P.L. 92-603, §§1161 et. seq.

36. Commerce Clearinghouse, "New Developments," *Medicare-Medicaid* 27, 456–27, 470 (see Transmittal 21).

37. Id. at 27, 456.

38. Id.

39. C. Steinwald, *An Introduction to Foundations for Medical Care,* (Chicago: Blue Cross, 1971).

40. Bryant, O'Donoghue, Toerber, *Current Perceptions by the Health Care Community of the Activities of Four Western Foundations for Medical Care* (Denver: Spectrum Research, 1975).

41. Id.

42. John Gilbert, *Preliminary Report* (On CHAMP) (Boston: Commonwealth Institute of Medicine, 1976).

43. Sanazaro, Goldstein, et al., "Research and Development in Quality Assurance, The Experimental Medical Care Review Organization," *New England Journal of Medicine* 287 (1972): 1125.

44. Goldstein, Roberts, et al., "Data for Peer Review: Acquisition and Use, Results in the Experimental Care Review Organization Program," *Annals of Internal Medicine* 82 (1975): 262.

45. Arthur D. Little, *Evaluation of the Hawaii EMCRO* (Cambridge: Arthur D. Little, 1974). See also, Goldstein, Id.

Chapter 2

The PSRO Law

THE PURPOSES OF THE LAW

PSRO is a comparatively new, and peculiarly limited, form of government-mandated medical peer review. The PSRO act itself states its purpose as follows:

> In order to promote the effective, efficient, and economical delivery of health care services of proper quality for which payment may be made [by Medicare or Medicaid] . . . and in recognition of the interests of patients, the public, practitioners, and providers in improved health care services, it is the purpose of this part to assure . . . that the services for which payment may be made . . . will conform to appropriate professional standards for the provision of health care and that payment for such services will be made—
> (1) only when, and to the extent, medically necessary . . .
> (2) in the case of services provided by a hospital or other health care facility . . . only when . . .
> Such services cannot, consistent with professionally recognized health care standards, effectively be provided on an outpatient basis or more economically. . . .[1]

But the official legislative history does not immediately consider "effectiveness." The opening paragraph of the Senate Finance Committee's justification for the law is:

> According to recent estimates the costs of the medicare hospital insurance program will overrun the estimates made in

19

1967, by some $240 billion over a 25-year period. The monthly premium costs for part B of medicare—doctor's bills—rose from a total of $6 monthly per person on July 1, 1966, to $11.60 per person on July 1, 1972. Medicaid costs are also rising at precipitous rates.

The report goes on to say:

In view of the per diem costs of hospital and nursing facility care, and the costs of medical and surgical procedures, the economic impact of this overutilization becomes extremely significant. Aside from the economic impact the committee is most concerned about the effect of overutilization on the health of the aged and the poor. Unnecessary hospitalization and unnecessary surgery are not consistent with proper health care.[2]

It is probably unfair to say that PSRO is "only a cost-control mechanism." Both the statute and the statutory history refer explicitly to quality-control problems: even in the statements of purpose, quoted above, one cannot help noticing the reliance on "appropriate professional standards," or the committee's concern, admittedly secondary to its financial concern, that overutilization harms patients.

There is visibly little concern with underutilization. Perhaps the committee felt that fear of malpractice litigation would keep physicians and hospitals from skimping on the provision of resources, but on this the record is silent.

What, then, should one say about the purpose of the PSRO law? Primarily, perhaps, that the statute was written to permit the government to cut, or at least limit the growth of, Medicare and Medicaid costs without forcing medical standards below an acceptable level.

The question then becomes: what mechanism has the law established with which to carry out its purpose?

BECOMING A PSRO

Between Congressional enactment and a program's full functioning, there necessarily exists a period in which regulations are drafted and redrafted, political compromises are made and people involved in the process try to meet Congressional goals without overrunning Congressional appropriations. In the case of the PSRO program, the anticipated political problems[3] were compounded by practical problems, some of which were obviously[4] not anticipated. Aside from funding cutbacks, the most serious problems may have been that, although all aspects of legislatively-mandated peer review had been suggested, tried, or successfully run somewhere in the country, no area or organization had successfully implemented all those activities simultaneously. From HEW's point of view, it must have looked like an awesome task of bringing dozens of separate review groups into existence or into the program. From the peer review groups' point of view, the problem must have been seen as one of coping with or changing hundreds of new federal regulations. And from the point of view of the physicians and other providers who wanted to participate but were not sure how to go about it, it was clearly a matter of getting whatever help was offered.

It is to the credit of all parties that a method of making the Congressional theory a reality was developed and implemented under the circumstances. Yet it must be acknowledged that faults in the method exist and may yet destroy the program. The remainder of this chapter will explore the way in which the PSRO program has been implemented, primarily from the perspective of the PSRO or would-be PSRO. Chapter 3 will examine the program's faults and alleged faults. Subsequent chapters will deal with the legal implications of various implementation options, some of which are likely to trouble PSROs and some of which are not. Chapter 9 will discuss how well the PSRO program has functioned so far, whether it can succeed, and the alternatives.

Regarding implementation, the steps by which a PSRO assumes operational responsibility are, broadly, the following:

Area Designation

Section 1152(a) commands HEW to "not later than January 1, 1974, establish . . . areas with respect to which [PSROS] may be designated. . . ." HEW must then enter into a contract with a "qualified organization" in each area, designating that organization as a conditional PSRO. Until the PSRO law was amended by PL 94-182, the sparse instructions in §1152(a) were the sum total of instructions from Congress to HEW on area designation. The legislative history which accompanied the statute was slightly more explicit, but, of course, is not binding.[5] The Committee report says, "In smaller or more sparsely populated states, the designation would probably be on a statewide basis. Each area, defined in geographic or medical service area terms, would generally include a minimum of 300 practicing physicians . . . It is expected that there will be many multi-county PSRO areas."[6]

Relying in large part on this nonbinding instruction from Congress, HEW formulated a policy which mandated that there be at least 300 physicians per PSRO area, at least 50,000 persons per PSRO area, and that no PSRO area cross a state line.[7] In cases where there were not enough physicians or patients in an entire state to constitute a minimum-size PSRO area, the state itself served as the PSRO boundary.

In some cases this has resulted in a given medical service area being cut up into two or more PSROs. For example, the greater New York medical service delivery area encompasses not only New York City and parts of New York State, but some of western Connecticut and parts of northern New Jersey. Albany's medical service area includes part of western Massachusetts; St. Louis's area covers part of southern Illinois. Examples of such regions exist wherever a major city is on or near a state border. This splitting up of service areas does not, it should be said, make the PSRO program, Medicare, or Medicaid any more difficult to handle administratively; the problem, basically, is that a given provider may have two different sets of criteria applying to different segments of its patient population. While Medicare may be willing to accept the review decision of any PSRO, Medicaid may not; Medicaid money is raised in part from state rather than federal taxes, and each state Medicaid agency will have a contractual arrangement with a limited number of PSROs, and no others. Hospitals which are near state boundaries and which accept patients from more than one Medicaid payer may have to do review under two sets of criteria or risk losing reimbursement because one or more of the involved PSROs have no alternative but to insist on the criteria which were not used.

This can be demonstrated by a simple hypothetical example. Suppose that the PSRO which covers Albany and the surrounding areas of New York State decides that a colectomy should be given five days of postoperative hospitalization before review for length-of-stay is indicated; suppose also that the Western Massachusetts PSRO decides that four days post-operative stay is all that is indicated. Now, suppose that a Medicaid patient from western Massachusetts is hospitalized in Albany for a colectomy, and that the reviewer in the Albany hospital, following the Albany PSRO guidelines, reviews the length-of-stay after five days. When the PSRO which is responsible for reviewing that patient's care for that patient's Medicaid payer, i.e., the Western Massachusetts PSRO, looks at the patient's PSRO record, it will be forced to decide that at least one day's care should not be reimbursed.

While the no-crossing-of-state-boundaries rule elicited some comment within the medical industry when HEW's area designation guidelines were first promulgated, it was a somewhat different problem which led to the first litigation on the law's area-designation provisions, and which, as a result, also led to the first amendment of that process. It is clear from a reading of both the statute and the guidelines that fifty single-state PSROs would not be impossible. It is probably fair to say that HEW has taken the position that it would designate the smallest possible PSROs within the 300-physician guideline. Some physicians' organizations have taken the position that HEW should have, rather, designated the largest possible PSROs within the guidelines. One such organization, the Texas Medical Association, went so far as to sue HEW for arbitrary, unreasonable, and capricious behavior in its failure to designate the entire state of Texas as a PSRO, and a federal trial judge agreed with them.[8]

In response to the lawsuit, a subsection (g) has been added to §1152 of the Social Security Act. This new subsection provides that, with the exception noted below, whenever HEW has designated two or more PSRO areas within a state, it must poll the state's physicians on the question, "Do you support a change from the present local and regional (PSRO) area designations to a single statewide area designation?" If 50% of the doctors in *each* previously-designated area of the state vote "yes," then HEW is required to designate the entire state as a PSRO area. This requirement does not apply in any state where HEW had already signed agreements with a conditional or fully operational PSRO prior to December 31, 1975, the date of the amendment's enactment.

The new subsection demonstrates a balance between HEW's desire to keep PSRO areas small, and presumably more manageable, and Congress's unwillingness to force a legal or political confrontation over what the Senate Finance Committee report tactfully described as "widespread physician concern over their inability to establish a single statewide PSRO..."[9] While the amendment at first appears to give the Texas Medical Association the statewide referendum that they demand, a sufficiently well-organized anti-statewide group of physicians could, by concentrating their efforts on a single previously designated PSRO area and winning there, defeat the pro-statewide physicians in the rest of the state.[10]

The RFP: Responding to HEW

Section 1152 (b) of the statute provides that for an organization to be considered qualified to become a PSRO it must be (1) a nonprofit, or part of a nonprofit, organization; (2) composed of M.D.s and/or D.O.s, representative of the area's physicians; (3) organized so that all necessary professional competences will be available for review; (4) voluntary and not limited to dues-paying members of the local or state medical society or other medical association; and (5) not internally discriminatory as regards eligibility to do review. Section 1152(b)(1)(B) then says that any other "public, nonprofit, or other" agency or organization may also be a qualified organization if the Secretary so determines, but §1152(c) prohibits HEW from contracting with such "other" qualified organization until after January 1, 1976 or 1978.

The deadlines exist simultaneously because §108 of PL 94-182 provides, in part, that the 1976 deadline specified in PL 92-603 be moved to January 1, 1978, except where the physicians in the PSRO area, or in the state in which the PSRO area is located, have taken a formal position "adopted by resolution or other official procedure or formal policy"[11] in opposition to the PSRO program, or where the Secretary of HEW has previously attempted to enter into a contract with an organization which would qualify under §1152(b)(1)(A) and has had that contract voted down by the area's physicians.

The reasons for the two exceptions, although they do not appear in any committee report, are not hard to imagine. It would be pointless to extend the deadline for physician control of the program in any area of the country where the physicians have gone on record as being committed to its opposition; and HEW may be entitled to look at the widest possible selection of applicant organizations if the first (physicians') group which has tried to become a PSRO has failed. This would be as true where the negative vote reflected antiprogram sentiment as it would where the vote reflected mere distrust of, or dissatisfaction with, the local applicant group. Polling and voting procedures will be considered in the next section.

In most areas of the country, PL 94-182's deferral of the deadline has enabled would-be PSROs to concentrate once again on meeting HEW's organizational requirements without fear that some "outside" (e.g., nonphysician) group will emerge to challenge their bid for federal funds.

Section 1152(b)(2) requires that HEW may not contract with a "qualified organization" as defined above (non-profit, representative, voluntary, etc.) unless HEW is also able, "on the basis of ... examination and evaluation of a formal plan" submitted to it by the would-be PSRO, to determine that the organization is "willing to perform and capable of performing, in an effective, timely, and objective manner and at reasonable cost, the duties, functions, and activities"[12] of a PSRO. The most logical reading of §1152(b)(2) is that an operational PSRO must actually be performing all of the duties required in sections 1155, 1156, 1157, 1160(b) and (c), 1161, and 1166. This reading is reinforced by the presence in the statute of §1154 ("Trial Period for Professional Standards Review Associations"), which creates the "conditional" PSRO, and §1152(a), which permits HEW to contract with such organizations to permit them to perform review.

An organization which has been "[designated] as a [PSRO]...on a conditional basis"[13] must submit to HEW "a formal plan for the orderly assumption and implementation"[14] of full statutory responsibilities during its "trial period"[15] and then implement its plan. The trial period may last no longer than 2 years (24 months),[16] at the end of which time the conditional PSRO must be fully operational or risk losing its federal funding.[17]

As those who have read the statute will have noticed, nowhere does the Congressional enactment or its legislative history contemplate the existence of such an organization as a "planning" PSRO. Nevertheless, as there were few organizations capable of performing the full scope of PSRO duties within two years, and as HEW was under some pressure from Congress to get the program started within a reasonable time after enactment, something had to be done. What HEW did was to develop the concept of the "planning" PSRO to permit it to allocate funds to nonprofit, voluntary physicians' organizations which were willing to perform such duties if given the time to develop the capabilities, and which HEW judged, on the basis of the evidence (proposals and site visits), that a period of intensive help might bring to the point where they could submit a plan which would qualify them under §1154 as "conditional" PSROs.

In order to elicit from potentially interested organizations information that would enable HEW to determine whether they "qualified" under subsections 1152(b) and (c), §1154, or the "planning" quasi regulations, HEW, like any government contractor, published and occasionally republishes a Request For Proposals (RFP) notice in the *Commerce Business Daily,* the federal publication for government contractors. Interested organizations are usually given 30 days to write for the RFP, read it, and respond, after which HEW evaluates the proposals, and, if necessary, makes a choice between two or more potential competing PSROs.[18]

In general, the RFPs have held strictly to the statutory requirements, striking new ground only where Congress left terms clearly undefined. For example, where §1152(b)(1)(A)(iii) says that a PSRO's membership shall include "a substantial proportion" of the licensed MDs and DOs in the PSRO's designated area, HEW's first "conditional" RFP required a minimum membership of 25% of those qualified to join. The only instance in which HEW appears to have exceeded its Congressional mandate is in its interpretation of §1152(b)'s requirement that PSROs shall be "organizations," a term of no special legal significance. HEW has chosen to demand that they incorporate (§§402.1 and 505.2 of the PSRO Program Manual require that a PSRO be a corporation, and §505.3 requires the corporation be not-for-profit, and the respective planning and conditional RFPs follow suit), although, speaking strictly, the PSRO statute appears to allow partnerships as an acceptable organizational form[19]. As it is HEW rather than Congress that administers the program, all PSROs have incorporated themselves in accordance with the laws of their several states, and applied for federal tax exemptions as nonprofit corporations.[20]

In most respects, RFPs have tended to echo statutory requirements quite closely. A fuller discussion of RFPs, contracts, and nonstatutory requirements can be found in Section 4 of this chapter.

Polling: Enlisting Physician Support

After area designation, and simultaneously with or immediately following the RFP response, the groups seeking PSRO contracts must enlist membership and ask for nonmember physician support. Both requirements derive from the statute: the membership enrollment requirement from §1152(b), as just discussed; and the support requirement from §1152(f), which provides that if, after notice, 10% of the physicians in the applicant's designated area object to the planned contract award, HEW must conduct a poll of all eligible area physicians to determine whether a majority of those who respond favor or object to the would-be PSROs being treated officially as their representative.

The PSRO statute does not establish specific enrollment procedures, and gives only the bare outlines of the notification and polling procedures. In fact, enrollment procedures remain undefined at the present time. Polling procedures, on the other hand, were established by HEW in 1974.[21] Under the regulations promulgated at that time, the entire burden of determining who is eligible to vote, notifying them, and conducting the poll, if necessary, rests on HEW. The PSRO applicant's only obligation is to try to persuade area physicians to support its continued existence. In most cases, those organizations which have been well-organized enough to receive favorable responses to their proposals from HEW have also been able to enlist the required 50% physician support. HEW's regulations neither deviate from nor significantly expand upon §1152(f), except for the provision in 42 CFR 101.107(c) that only one recount of any poll will be allowed, although a written request from any five involved physicians will precipitate that recount. (42 CFR 101.106(c) does provide that ballots will be available for public inspection at least until the 10-day recount request period has run out.)

PSROs IN OPERATION

For the purpose of analyzing the law as it applies to the operational PSRO, it seems best to look at the statute's commands and permissions as they affect the PSRO's major routine functions. Accordingly, this section will deal with the following six areas:

- reviewing (including data-gathering)
- delegation
- reporting
- sanctions
- payment
- interactons with Medicare and Medicaid.

In each of these areas, the statute's minimum requirements and allowable options will be outlined.

Reviewing

The statutory sections that deal with the PSRO's primary function—the reviewing of medical care—are §1155(a) thru (d), and §1156.

Scope of Review

Section 1155(a) (1) says that the PSRO must review all institutional services provided by physicians and other health care providers, including institutional providers. The PSRO may review noninstitutional services, although subsection (g) of §1155 provides that review of noninstitutional services shall not be performed until HEW has given its approval to the PSRO's noninstitutional-care review plan. In reviewing any of these services, the PSRO must determine whether the services are medically necessary, of the quality which meets professionally recognized standards of health care, and are provided in the least expensive facility "consistent with the provision of appropriate medical care."[22] These three tests are known as the tests of necessity, quality, and appropriateness, and shall be so designated in the following discussion.

Review Methodology: Content

Section 1156(a) requires each PSRO to "apply professionally developed norms of care, diagnosis, and treatment based upon typical patterns of practice in its regions (including typical lengths-of-stay ... by age and diagnosis)." If, however, the PSRO develops norms significantly different from those developed elsewhere, the PSRO can, after "appropriate consultation and discussion," be forced to use norms developed elsewhere and approved by the National Professional Standards Review Council.

In any discussion of the sanctity of regional norms, one must bear in mind §1156(a)'s requirements that the norms may, within regulatory limits, be varied to allow for difference in treatment modality or type of facility.

While the standards-development process is not fully elaborated in the statute, there is one caveat. The most logical possible reading of §1156(c)(1) is that no PSRO may use its own regionally developed norms, criteria, or standards until after the National Professional Standards Review Council (NPSRC) has approved them. It can therefore be argued that in the absence of such approval, review is, at best, not binding, and, at worst, not legal. It would also be possible to argue, on the basis of §1156(c)(1), that no PSRO can achieve conditional status until the National PSRC has approved at least some of its review criteria, especially as §1156(c)(2) would seem to indicate that review for necessity, quality, and appropriateness may not be based on any norms, criteria, or standards not developed through the §1156(c)(1) process, which includes NPSRC review and approval. Any PSRO decision (e.g., to recommend payment or denial of Medicare or Medicaid funds) which is based on a finding of compliance or noncompliance with nonapproved criteria is probably a void decision; and any grant of conditional status by HEW to a PSRO is arguably either void or illegal until the NPSRC has reviewed and approved at least some of the PSRO's criteria. If a court were to accept this line of reasoning, it would obviously make a difference in a case where statewide area designation is being sought under Section 1152(g) but where HEW and, formerly, the physicians involved believed the option to have been foreclosed by HEW's conditional designation of one or more PSROs in the state.

The only instances in which the "content" of the PSRO's review decision is not bound by PSRO-developed, NPSRC-approved norms, standards, and criteria are the "medical care evaluation" studies, or MCEs. These will be discussed below.

Review Methodology: Process

Section 1156(d) provides that each PSRO must require from each reviewed attending physician periodic concurrent certification that his patient still requires institutional care. Such certification may not be required any later than that day of stay on which fifty percent of patients of a similar age and with a similar diagnosis would have been discharged from the hospital. Section 1156(d), therefore, mandates that each PSRO must do concurrent utilization review substantially similar to the UR required under existing Medicare and Medicaid regulations.

Subsection 1152(a)(2) permits, but does not require, PSROs to do what is known as preadmission screening. The statutory language is that each PSRO "shall have the authority" to determine in advance the reimbursability of any elective admission or admission for extended or costly course of treatment.

For the posture of future litigation it is crucial that preadmission screening not be required. If the logic of *AMA v. Weinberger*[23] (a case which will be discussed in Chapter 4), is followed, HEW may never be permitted to actually require that preadmission screening be performed. This leaves any PSRO which wishes to perform such preadmission screening in an exposed legal position, as the PSRO could be attacked for arbitrariness, capriciousness, and unconstitutionality in requiring a type of screening which HEW may itself be prohibited from making mandatory. It should be noted that the legal questionability of §1152(a)(2) would not necessarily taint concurrent admission screening performed under the authority of §1156(d), although the *AMA v. Weinberger* court did not distinguish between admission (concurrent) and preadmission screening. In many jurisdictions, a patient's right to treatment at a given facility depends on whether the patient has been admitted or not. In such places, the distinction between preadmission and postadmission screening may materially affect the patient's chance to be seen by a physician.

Section 1155(a)(3) requires each PSRO to publish a list of the types of cases or diseases for which it will do the preadmission screening permitted in §1155(a)(2). If §1155(a)(2) becomes impossible for a PSRO to carry out, §1155(a)(3) will become a dead letter; if, by chance, some PSROs do manage to do preadmission screening, §1155(a)(3) will require them to notify the physicians in their areas of those types of nonemergency cases which will be subjected to that type of screening.

Section 1155(a)(4) requires every PSRO to arrange and maintain "profiles" for each patient, practitioner, and provider covered by the program. "Profiles shall ... be regularly reviewed ... to determine whether the care and services ordered or rendered are consistent with the criteria ..." of necessity, quality and appropriateness. The section may contain a hidden agenda: while it is understandable that review of practitioners' and providers' profiles could help the PSRO discover unnecessary, inappropriate, or poor quality care, it is less clear—although certainly not impossible—that review of patients' profiles will lead to any of the three stated goals. What is more likely is that patient profile review will unmask patients who are "abusing" the medical system—and the third-party payors—by seeing several practitioners simultaneously for the same complaint, or by obtaining admission to multiple facilities and therefore receiving unnecessary diagnostic workups, when a single admission, or readmission to a single facility, would be sufficient.

It is only fair to say that review of a patient's profile may permit the PSRO to discover quality-of-care problems (e.g., prescription of a medication which reacts unfavorably with other medications taken by the patient without the prescribing doctor's knowledge) or medical-necessity problems (e.g., overfrequent hospital admissions) which would not necessarily be apparent from the review of any single chart belonging to that patient. Whether or not the PSRO could take effective action to halt a patient's abuse of the system is subject to some speculation, given the unsettled state of the law of privacy in the PSRO context and given the PSRO's legal duty to refrain from arbitrarily penalizing the honestly ignorant providers or practitioners who care for such patients.

Medical Care Evaluation studies, which are retrospective[24] and/or concurrent reviews of patients' charts (and/or patient, practitioner, and/or provider profiles) in order to develop standards or assess quality, are mentioned nowhere in PL 92-603's §249F. It is not clear that Congress contemplated that PSROs would become involved in medical audit, which is, of course, the pre-HEW name for at least one type of MCE. The legislative history is silent on the point, with the single possible exception of the following statement in the Senate Finance Committee report:

> ... The review process would be made more sophisticated through the use of professionally developed ... norms of diagnosis and care as guidelines for review ... The present review process ... becomes ... episodic [and] subjective ...[25]

It seems probable, however, that Congress was not aware of the criteria-development or quality-monitoring aspects of medical audit when that statement was made, because immediately afterwards the Finance Committee report continues:

> ... The present review process ... [fails] to take into account in a systematic fashion the experience gained through past reviews or to sufficiently emphasize general findings about the pattern of care provided.[26]

This is profile review, not chart-based medical audit. It is therefore questionable whether HEW has the authority to appropriate federal funds for MCE studies, and it is just as unclear whether or not PSROs can legally require that hospitals perform MCEs as a condition of being delegated the authority to do review.

Having said all that, however, one must nevertheless admit that judicious use of MCEs, as the concept of medical audit has been formulated by HEW, can be of enormous utility to any PSRO which is sincerely interested in the development of standards.[27] The fact remains that there must be some way for the PSRO to document the basis on which nonsubjective peer decisions are made, and the MCE can help define the reviewers' reasons for setting their limits at one level rather than another. To deprive the reviewers of this tool would, to some extent, vitiate §1155(c)'s implied promise that rational professional judgment can be exercised by peer reviewers within the program, and in fact to negate the entire need for professional input into PSROs. Norms cannot be "professionally developed;"[28] they are generated by observed behavior. In a very real sense, the difference between a quality "norm" and a quality "standard" is the difference between average practice and the range of practices desired by, or at least acceptable to, an impartial group of physicians. To limit the PSROs' peer reviewers to judging quality of care solely against norms is to risk locking the PSRO program into paying for average care even when that average is demonstrably unsatisfactory.

Furthermore, it is hard to argue that the statute's failure to mention MCEs or any other form of medical audit must be taken as a repudiation of the method, even though the legislative history seems clearly to indicate that the technique was not contemplated by those who drafted and voted on the measure. This is especially true where later legislative history shows no Congressional objections to the uses of MCEs which had, by then, been suggested by HEW. It is possible to say that medical quality audit, in the form of the MCE, has become a part of the PSRO review process, and its required use could possibly be upheld by a court if attacked. Whether it would in fact be upheld is another matter, especially in view of the continued absence of regulations mandating its use.

It might be wise at this point to stop to examine again the review system which the PSRO law appears to contemplate in regard to Medicare and Medicaid patients. Preadmission and retrospective review are permissible, but not required. Concurrent review, at least for utilization (i.e., necessity and appropriateness), is required. Such review, whether concurrent, prospective, or retrospective, must be based on objective norms, standards, and criteria which have been "developed" by the PSRO and/or validated by the National PSRC.

Reviewers

Statutory language concerning the responsibilities of persons doing peer review is, for the most part, clear and unambiguous. Section 1155(a)(5) states that the PSRO may not assign any physician to review hospital services unless that physician has active staff privileges at no less than one PSRO-area hospital. If the PSRO is reviewing care provided by a "nondelegated" hospital, reviewing physicians with staff privileges in that hospital may "participate in . . . [but] should not be responsible for" that review. What this last requirement means in practice has yet to be determined. One possible way of handling the problem would be for the PSRO to say that physicians from a nondelegated hospital may not be a majority of any group of physicians voting on any determination about care provided by that hospital.

Section 1155(a)(6) contains prohibitions against conflict of interest by reviewers. No physician shall be permitted to review "health care services provided to a patient if [the physician] was directly or indirectly involved in providing such services, or . . . health care services provided in or by [any facility] . . . if [the physician] or any member of his family has . . . any financial interest in that facility." The subsection also defines what members of the physician's family are included in the prohibition. It does *not* define what constitutes "financial interest." In a very real sense, every physician has a financial interest in the continued solvency of the institutions to which he admits patients. If, however, §1155(a)(6) were read that broadly, §1155(e), which permits delegation of review authority to hospital-based committees, would be void. A reading of §1155(a)(6) which avoids the conflict would interpret "financial interest" as equivalent to an ownership interest.[29] This reading would permanently exclude the physician-owners of proprietary hospitals from serving on their own UR/PSRO committees whenever the proprietary hospital was seeking delegated status. Although it is not legally required, a PSRO might decide to presume that no small proprietary hospital should be delegated even then, given the very real conflict-of-interest possibilities. Whether such a presumption could be made binding is, of course, open to question.[30]

Section 1155(b)(1) permits PSROs to utilize nonphysicians to help review nonphysician care. While some nonphysician provider organizations have interpreted this section to require the PSRO to utilize the services of, e.g., dentists or nurses in reviewing, respectively, reimbursable dental or nursing care, such a reading is probably overbroad, given the statutory statement that the PSRO is "authorized" to utilize such services but is nowhere "required" to utilize such services. It should also be noted that the input of such other medical practitioners will be at best advisory, as §1155(a)(1) requires the PSRO as a whole to be the ultimate determiner of the necessity, quality, and appropriateness of all covered services, and as §1152(b) requires that, until HEW says otherwise, PSROs shall be composed entirely of M.D.s and D.O.s. It is not clear that a PSRO could legally contract to be bound by the vote of nonphysicians reviewing nonphysician care. On the other hand, it is also probable that a PSRO's refusal to at least accept such advisory opinions might be considered arbitrary, unreasonable, and capricious, as PSRO members will ordinarily lack the educational or experiential backgrounds to make judgments about services outside their field.

As is true in other areas, the Finance Committee report here is more forceful than the statute it seeks to explicate. In regard to §1155(b)(1), the legislative history states that "it is expected" that PSROs would make specific arrangements with groups representing substantial numbers of dentists for necessary review of dental services. "PSROs would ... be expected to retain and consult with other types of health care practitioners such as podiatrists to assist in reviewing ..."[31] There is a difference between "authorized," "expected," and "required," and it will ultimately be up to HEW, by its regulations, and the courts, to determine which reading of §1155(b)(1) is factually to be the most accurate.[32]

Section 1155(c) states explicitly that no "final determination" of any review decision shall be made by anyone other than an M.D. or D.O. if the care involved was provided by an M.D. or D.O. Given the all-physician composition of the PSRO, and its total authority for reviewing, §1155(c) might seem to be redundant. However, there may come a time, sometime after January 1, 1978, when HEW sees fit to designate a nonphysician group as an area PSRO. In such a case, §1155(c) would still protect physicians from having nonphysicians review their care.

Section 1155(d) requires each PSRO to solicit physicians to participate as reviewers, rotate physician membership on review committees, make committees as broadly representative as possible of area specialities or types of practice, and report on their activities in local medical periodicals and "similar publications."

Delegation

Section 1155(e) requires PSROs to "utilize the services of, and accept findings of, the review committees of a hospital ... or organization located in the area served by (the PSRO), but only when ... such commit-

tees ... have demonstrated ... their capacity ... to review activities ... so as to aid in accomplishing the purposes and responsibilities
described in subsection (a)(1), except where the Secretary disapproves,
for good cause, such acceptance." Section 1155(e)(2) permits but does
not require HEW to prescribe regulations in regard to this subsection.

This section, known as the delegation section, permits PSROs to delegate to hospitals, other institutions, and/or HMOs, the responsibility for
reviewing the care provided within their jurisdictions for necessity,
quality, and appropriateness. Certain financial and legal considerations
have made this paragraph assume considerable significance to many institutional providers, and these considerations will be discussed in the
section on reimbursement in this chapter and in Chapter 3. It is a measure of the seriousness of the delegation issue that, in at least one case, a
PSRO has been sued by a hospital for failure to delegate review authority. (The suit was withdrawn when the PSRO made the delegation
rather than go to court.)

As of this writing, HEW has not enacted any regulations under
§1155(e); PSROs are largely left to their own devices in establishing delegation criteria. HEW has "suggested," in transmittals and in the PSRO
Program Manual, a six-step recommended delegation process intended
to lead to PSRO-hospital "Memoranda of Understanding." If followed,
this process will generate copious documentation of the PSRO's internal
decision-making procedures. Such documentation, one supposes, could
serve either to convince HEW to approve the PSRO's delegation decisions or to persuade a judge or jury of the essential rationality and
nonarbitrariness of those same decisions. These transmittals will be discussed in somewhat greater detail near the end of this chapter. The
transmittals' "suggestions" have recently been formalized as proposed
rules 42 CFR 101.804–101.807, 101.809, and 101.810.

It should be noted that "partial delegation," some forms of which are
allowed by HEW, is neither permitted nor prohibited by §1155(e). The
statute speaks only of review committee results, and does not concern
itself with review coordinators. The distinction has not been very important, as HEW and many PSROs have taken the position that, coordinators' decisions being nondiscretionary (anything falling within PSRO-
established norms must be approved; anything falling outside must be
referred "upstairs" for individual and/or committee peer review), coordinator performance will be deemed inextricably linked to committee
performance. It should be obvious, however, that a hospital seeking delegation can have superb coordinators and a self-serving committee, lazy
or inaccurate coordinators and a good committee, or any other possible
combination, and that bad coordinators can sabotage a hospital's efforts

to meet PSRO standards as effectively as can a slack or self-serving internal peer review committee.[33]

Some PSROs, especially in Western states, have recognized the distinction between coordinator performance and committee performance. They have indicated their willingness—in fact, their desire—to "partially delegate" review authority to hospitals, so that the PSRO would train, employ, and monitor the coordinators, while the delegated hospitals' previously established review committees would continue to make those review decisions which call for the exercise of medical judgment. Under §1155(e) it would be equally possible, although there are no practical examples, for a PSRO to permit the hospitals to hire and train coordinators while the PSRO's peer reviewers judged the nonroutine cases. It appears, however, that even those PSROs which are willing to attempt full delegation are not willing to let hospitals with nondelegated committees control the coordinators.

Reporting and Confidentiality

The PSRO statute contains a number of reporting requirements, one of which—§1156(c)'s requirement that proposed norms, criteria, and standards be reported to the National PSRC—has been discussed. The most crucial of these reporting requirements is §1157's absolute mandate that violations of §1160 be reported to the statewide PSR Council, which must then report the case to HEW.

The crucial section of §1160 is its subsection (a), which, basically, makes it the legal obligation of every practitioner or provider to render services only when medically necessary. These services must be of acceptable quality and provided "in such form and fashion and at such time as may be reasonably required" by the PSRO. These requirements parallel those in §1155(a). Section 1160(a)(2) further requires that no provider or practitioner may take "any action . . . which would authorize any individual to be admitted as an inpatient" or maintain inpatient status unless the health care provided is necessary and provided in the least expensive appropriate facility.

When the requirements of §1160 are read back into §1157, it becomes clear that any discrepancy between a practitioner's practice and any applicable PSRO norm, criterion, or standard is reportable to HEW via the statewide PSRC.[34] This does not, of course, require the PSRO or the state PSRC to take disciplinary action or apply any type of sanction. It does mean, however, that the information will be on file with a federal agency, subject to whatever disclosure rules that agency may promulgate within the law. No matter how lenient or stringent an individual

PSRO's confidentiality policy may be, it cannot affect HEW's own rules regarding the data it has been given. A fuller discussion of this problem can be found in Chapter 6.

Section 1159 provides that the PSRO must notify all affected persons (patients, providers, and/or practitioners) of adverse determinations, such as no-pay decisions, of any cases reviewed. Any aggrieved patient, provider, or practitioner may ask for a "reconsideration" by the PSRO of its initial decision; where the amount in controversy is $100.00 or more, the reconsideration is subject to automatic review by the state PSRC, in states where a PSRC exists. The aggrieved party is also entitled to go to a hearing before HEW if the case involves $100.00 or more, and to judicial review if the case involves $1000.00 or more. While §1159 of the statute does not specify what types of notices and reports must be submitted during the course of such hearings, reconsiderations, and appeals, the matter has been dealt with to some extent by regulations which appeared in the *Federal Register* on February 20, 1976.[35] These regulations applied to such cases the hearings and appeals procedures under Title XVIII, Part A, of the Social Security Act.

Section 1160(b)(1) deals with HEW's ability to "exclude (permanently [or] for such period as the Secretary may prescribe) [a] practitioner or provider from eligibility to provide ... services on a reimbursable basis" if he or it fails "in a substantial number of cases substantially to comply with any obligation imposed" to provide only necessary and appropriate services, or has "grossly and flagrantly [violated that] obligation in one or more instances." This section does not require that the PSRO involved provide special notice of any sort. Rather, the notice requirement appears to rest on HEW itself. This is certainly true in §1160(b)(1), which cannot be read otherwise without creating a conflict with the mandatory language of §1157 ("[the] organization shall report"), so that the grammatical subject of §1160(b)(1) is "he", i.e., the Secretary of HEW, and the verb is "may exclude." Similarly, the notice requirements in Section 1160(b)(2) and (b)(4) can only be read as being the responsibility of HEW and not of the involved PSRO.

What reporting and/or confidentiality rules will apply to any PSRO in its effort to comply with §1160(c) are, at the moment, even more open to speculation. Section 1160(c) requires PSROs and PSRCs to use their "authority or influence" to enlist the influence or support of other professional or government agencies to enforce practitioner and provider compliance with §1160(a). It is difficult, although clearly not impossible, to imagine how a PSRO or PSRC could enlist such support without explaining to the involved professional or governmental organization just what kinds of infraction they are seeking support in helping to erase.

How this can be done without also involving, at least to some extent, the "who" is a problem which has not yet received much attention, but which could prove to be as difficult as any of the confidentiality problems yet encountered by PSROs.

Section 1161 of the PSRO law reinforces §1159(a)'s requirement that notice be given whenever the PSRO has made an adverse determination; §1161 also requires that a PSRO give notice to any provider or practitioner when it feels there has been a violation of a §1160 obligation. This last requirement would probably be enforced, even in the absence of statutory section 1161, as a result of §1157's requirement that such determinations must be reported to HEW in all cases. To make such reports, which would have severe consequences under §1160(b), without notification would probably be a denial of due process of law; due process at the very least means that any person who may be subject to a government sanction as a result of an agency's adjudicatory proceeding has at least the same fundamental rights as an accused subject in a court proceeding which could result in a similarly severe sanction.

Having determined that the PSRO must make several kinds of reports to its various higher authorities, what protection does the individual patient, provider, or practitioner have against indiscriminate disclosure of information which could be acutely embarrassing or financially harmful? The confidentiality requirements of the PSRO law are set forth in §§1166 and 1167 of the statute. While §1166(a)(1) clearly permits all disclosures required by all previous sections of the PSRO statute, §1166(a)(2) allows HEW to provide regulations which "assure adequate protection of the rights and interests of patients, health care practitioners, or providers of health care" in determining what further revelations, if any, will be permitted. If any person discloses data or information acquired by any PSRO for any purpose other than those permitted by statute or regulation, such person "shall, upon conviction, be fined not more than $1,000, and imprisoned not more than six months, or both, together with the costs of prosecution."[36] While the official legislative history is silent on this point, it is probable that Congress intended the $1,000 or six months to be a significant deterrent to unpermitted disclosures.

Section 1155(a)(4), in addition to requiring that profiles be made, requires that "to the greatest extent practicable . . . methods of coding which will provide maximum confidentiality as to patient identity and assure objective evaluation" shall be used. Since a more stringent requirement ("shall not be disclosed" except as listed) of confidentiality can be found in §1166, which deals with data or information acquired by a PSRO, a logical reading of the statute is that material generated by a

PSRO need not be as stringently protected as the raw information supplied to a PSRO. There is, of course, an alternate reading. It is possible that §1155(a)(4)'s special protection of patients' confidentiality, as opposed to §1166's protection of patient, provider, and practitioner confidentiality, is meant not to apply to release of such data outside the PSRO, but, rather, is designed to deal only with internal use of the data. Under such a reading, §1155(a)(4)'s protection of patient-identifiable data would be meant only to keep internal review from being biased. As the legislative history is silent as to which is the correct reading, the matter will probably be determined by litigation.

Section 1155(f) requires PSROs to collect data and keep records in a format which will permit access to and use of such records by HEW. The most logical reading of §1155(f)(1)(b) is that such record keeping requirements will be developed in the HEW-PSRO contract and therefore need not be subject to the regulations process. If this is the correct reading, it conflicts, to some extent, with §1166's requirement that HEW shall use the regulatory process to solve problems of data confidentiality. While it might be possible to resolve the ambiguity by reading §1155(f) to deal with financial and organizational records of the PSRO rather than with its review records, such a reading is not explicitly justified by any limitation within §1155(f) itself.

Section 1167, while not dealing with disclosure by a PSRO or the confidentiality required of a PSRO, does create what is known as a "privilege" for information imparted to a PSRO by any person. While this basically permits reports to be made to a PSRO, it does not apply any special duties on the organization.

Sanctions

At first glance, the PSRO statute appears to limit PSROs, unlike private peer-review organizations, to two sanctioning procedures: denying reimbursement (§1158), and reporting errant providers to HEW (§1160(b)). A more correct reading, however, is that these two procedures are the only two which are mandatory, and that PSROs have the option, under §1160(c), of using the whole range of educational and disciplinary processes which are available to the purely private organizations.

For the purpose of this discussion of sanctions, it should be assumed that the PSRO or other peer review group has, through review, not only discovered that there is a discrepancy between its standard(s) and the care which was, or is being, rendered, but also that the discrepancy results from suboptimal care. It cannot be overstressed, especially in situations where screening criteria are untried or unsophisticated, that deviation from the norm will not always indicate a need for correction or discipline.

Consider the following example: Dr. Jones and Dr. Smith, both internists who admit patients to Downtown General Hospital, are reviewed by Region 225 PSRO, whose computer reveals that both have exceeded length-of-stay norms an average of 15 days on 34% of their patients. This information is handed to the Region 225 PSRO peer review panel, which, after suitable review, discovers that Dr. Jones' patients seem to exceed their LOS norms because they suffer numerous complications, the reasons for which cannot be ascertained because of a near-total absence of progress notes in Dr. Jones' charts. Dr. Smith's patients, however, clearly exceed their LOS norms because they are generally elderly and recover slowly from their acute illnesses, often because (as Dr. Smith's progress notes reflect) they are also suffering from two or more unrelated chronic illnesses of varying severity. Dr. Jones would be a candidate for the imposition of some sanction; Dr. Smith would not. If the nurses' notes reveal that Dr. Jones' inadequate charting reflects a real neglect of his patients, the sanction might be more severe than it would if the nurses' notes show that he was attentive but unwilling to admit that certain symptoms were likely to be the precursors of certain other complications.[37]

The point of this example is, obviously, that appropriate action by a PSRO, hospital, or other peer review organization will depend not only on the degree to which norms are exceeded or standards violated, but also on the reasons for the excess or violation. With that caveat in mind, it should be possible to deal with the sanctions available to peer review organizations.

The following are some of the options which each PSRO or private peer review organization can consider in dealing with individual practitioners or institutions whose medical care is determined to be substandard or unjustifiably outside the norm:

Notification

The PSRO can notify the physician that his practice has been determined to fall repeatedly below acceptable norms and standards. No further action by the PSRO may need to be undertaken.

Simple notification may or may not influence physician practice patterns. It has been the experience of some Foundations for Medical Care that when a physician is notified of his substandard care, or even when he is simply asked to provide further information for review, he will make adequate efforts to improve his care and will seek advice in order to do so.[38] It has also been noted by FMCs that the simple publication of peer-set standards, norms and criteria (as the PSRO law specifically requires)[39] will encourage most physicians to adhere to them. Also, fairness to the physician (and the PSRO statute, in §1160(b)(1)) requires that notification, which has the advantage of being the simplest step, should be initiated as a first course of action whenever a more serious sanction is contemplated.

Tighter Review

The PSRO can place the physician or institution on closer peer review. This might mean that the PSRO would require preadmission certification and/or more frequent or more stringent concurrent review for the involved physician. Most commentators have concluded that retrospective review is inadequate to control the continually "deviant" provider, even though such providers may have first been identified by retrospective review.

Placing the physician "on review" is an option which the PSRO may have to take for its own protection in certain instances, as failure to do so could become (depending on future regulations) a violation of §1155(a)(2), but such a step could also encourage the affected practitioner to modify his practice and thereby help his patients. If such an improvement is documented, the PSRO can and probably should return the physician to routine review procedures, but may choose to monitor him intermittently to prevent backsliding.

When the hospital as a whole is put "on review" for some systemic impediment to the delivery of adequate care, the PSRO would obviously be well-advised to demand evidence of implementation of an appropriate remedy before the hospital is returned to routine screening status. It should also go without saying that if a PSRO finds that a delegated hospital is organizationally incapable of adequately handling certain types of patient problems, and that it has failed to initiate corrective action, it should be removed from delegated status. Review committees at delegated hospitals are the PSRO's agents, not buffers for the medical staff and administration.

Payment Denial

Section 1158(a) provides that if care is determined to be "unnecessary" or "inappropriate"[40] payment can and indeed must be withheld by the federal payors. The definitions of "unnecessary" and "inappropriate" are not necessarily medical definitions, and at least initially will depend, to some extent, on long-standing Medicaid and Medicare policies and limitations. The degree of correlation between a finding that care was "unnecessary" or that it was "inappropriate" and a finding that it did not meet standards for quality is, at present, not established. There may be little or no correlation between the findings; there may be a high correlation. In short, case-by-case peer review may result in "no-payment" decisions which have very little relevance to the quality of care. Medical care of high quality may not be covered under a given reimbursement program, and peer review, in such cases, may only highlight the differences between (or inadequacies of) certain benefit packages.

Education

The PSRO can recommend to the physicians (or to the hospital, for the benefit of itself and its nursing or administrative staff) or require that certain continuing education courses be taken. It can also suggest to, or require of, the physician certain educational remedies which would effectively demonstrate proper courses of medical care, such as attendance at grand rounds, going on ward rounds with a consultant, etc.[41]

Consultation

The PSRO can recommend or require that a physician obtain a consultant's aid on the next few cases of the type in question as a precondition for reimbursement. Many peer review groups report that they have found this to be an effective method of improving physicians' performance. Possibly this is because consultation is a standard practice and is accepted by most physicians; the consultant functions, in part, as an individual teacher whose recommendations can be measured by the physician in question against his own medical care decisions. The consultant can also refer the errant physician to pertinent medical literature and peer-based decisions in medical care.

Notification of HEW

Section 1160(b)(1) of the statute specifies that, while ordinarily single instances of unnecessary, substandard, or undocumented care should not be penalized, repeated instances should be, and single instances can be if there has been "gross" or "flagrant" violation of the section's prohibitions.

Penalties under §1160 will be assessable by HEW and not by the individual PSRO; but, as was discussed in the section on notifications, HEW cannot act until the PSRO asks it to do so and the PSRO has given appropriate notice to the provider (physician or hospital) and public. There are two possible penalties: (1) suspension or exclusion from eligibility for reimbursement or (2) a fine of up to $5000 or the cost of the unnecessary/improper services, whichever is less.

Reporting to Other Government or Private Agencies

The PSRO can submit the physician's name to his local medical or specialty society, report PSRO action to the hospital or long-term care facility in which the physician practices, or submit the physician's name to the appropriate state licensing authority or to the State PSR Council for remedial action. If the subject of the sanction is a hospital, the PSRO could notify the appropriate licensing or accrediting authority.

It should be stressed that these last options should be utilized *only* in the most severe cases. Overly frequent reliance by a peer review group on the "big guns" of publicity, licensure, accreditation, and censure will tend to make area medical professionals somewhat edgy; if the PSRO turns out to have been unjustified in its choice of a severe sanction with any frequency (e.g., more than once), their wariness is quite likely to deepen into overt hostility and noncooperation. It should be obvious, for instance, that submitting a physician's name to the local medical society or specialty society is a serious matter even though the local and specialty societies cannot impair the right to practice in any direct way.[42]

However, the societies can exert peer pressure on the individual physician if the members feel that it is indicated. Communication with the medical or specialty society can be especially useful if the PSRO has uncovered cases of probable malpractice, even when the errors have not resulted in harm to the patient(s). In such circumstances the society, if it decides to act by dropping or decertifying the individual practitioner, can be most effective.

Notification of the errant physician's hospital is probably the procedure of choice whenever the PSRO has clear evidence of fraud or malpractice and where actual or potential harm to patients would justify the hospital's taking disciplinary action. The advantage of choosing this option is that, among the disciplinary actions available to the hospital, selective suspension of practice privileges is an acceptable course; if it is chosen, those patients who would have been at risk can be protected while the physician may continue to be able to treat patients whom he would not harm.

Notifying the state medical licensure board is widely regarded as a less-than-fully-useful procedure, since state boards act slowly and are often bound by formal "trial-type" rules of evidence and procedure. However, state board procedures could become more responsive if

PSRO physician profiles become acceptable evidence[43] and if PSRO members in testifying can and do explain the profiles' meaning and significance on the witness stand. Some of the same problems—slowness of procedure and questions about the evidentiary value of PSRO findings —might plague the peer review group that reports a substandard hospital to the state board of hospital licensure or to national accrediting authorities, such as JCAH.

But before the PSRO arrives at the point at which it is willing to "go public" with its reports on the basis of §1160(c)'s permission, it should be remembered that all of these actions are subject to the important caveat that current HEW draft guidelines probably prohibit release of such information without the provider's prior approval. Unless the regulations differ substantially from the presently-available guidelines, none of the above steps is recommended; certainly none should be taken until after final regulations have been issued. This caveat does not apply to notifications sent to the State PSR Council or to HEW; the notifications are expressly permitted by §1157, which does not require provider permission for release of data. In all other cases, PSROs would probably be well advised to confine their remedial actions to those which operate internally.

All warnings about the legal and political undesirability of releasing information about sanctions outside the PSRO apply *a fortiori* to release to the public, including nonPSRO medical professionals. This is not to imply that consumers and other providers do not have a right to know about substandard doctors and hospitals—they very well may—or that such release might not have a salutary effect on deviant practitioners, but simply to say that to release such information in the absence of clear statutory or regulatory permission, or a court decision in favor of release, is to invite litigation.

If the PSRO or other peer review organization keeps within its written policy boundaries in applying sanctions, it should be able to avoid trouble.

In general, institutional quality problems may, but need not, be treated differently from physicians' problems. Although the severity of the initial corrective actions may differ in some respects between the two groups (PSROs may be likely to deny payment to a hospital where they would recommend some other procedure for a physician, such as consultation or continuing education), there is no statutory command that the same remedies be applied in all cases in which practice is found to be substandard. The only instances in which choice is denied to the PSRO are: (1) where facility use is unnecessary or inappropriate, in which cases payment must be denied; and (2) where the physician or institution is found to be in violation of §1160(a), in which case HEW or the State PSRC must be notified pursuant to §1157. In all other cases, §1160(c) would appear to give the PSRO nearly total freedom of action.

Reimbursement

As of this writing, no settled method of payment for PSRO review has yet been announced by HEW. Until quite recently, those conditional PSROs with sufficient budgets were reviewing; smaller conditionals and planning PSROs were waiting for the announcement and biding time. To undertand how the program had reached this impasse on the reimbursement question, it is necessary to consider the history of statutory sections 1168, 1815(b), and 1861(w).

In §1168, enacted by §249 F of PL 92-603, Congress provided that PSRO "expenses incurred ... shall be payable from—(a) funds in the Federal Hospital Insurance Trust Fund; (b) funds in the Federal Supplementary Medical Insurance Trust Fund; and (c) funds appropriated to carry out the health care provisions of the several divisions of the several titles of this Act; ...." It would hardly be possible for Congress to state more clearly that PSRO review was to be funded from Medicare and Medicaid as well as from direct appropriations. This reading of the law is reinforced by the legislative history, in which the Senate Finance Committee wrote (as part of a discussion of PSROs' right to do review for private insurers), "in such a case, there would be a proportionate allocation of costs between Medicare, Medicaid, and others served by the review organization."[44]

Had adequate (as judged by hospitals and PSROs actually performing or about to perform review) funding been available from one or more of the three sources named in §1168, review activities would presumably have begun as soon as HEW's approval of the several review plans was obtained. It is therefore probably unfortunate that initial PSRO appropriations were not sufficient to pay the cost of actually doing review in more than a handful of geographic areas.[45] Although it had initially been assumed by many that whoever did review would pay at least the direct costs of the review program, it soon became clear that, with the program as underfunded as it was, such a policy would create financial disincentives for review.

Hospitals were reluctant to assume the costs of reviewing, even in those increasingly rare areas of the country where costs can be passed directly on to the patients and third-party reviewers without prior governmental approval, because the hospitals could not be sure that review costs would be fully reimbursed. PSROs found themselves the recipients of lump sums of money which had to cover their entire operating costs, to which the actual reviewing of patients' records contributed one small part. It was therefore reasonable for the hosptials to ask the PSROs to pay for review, just as it was reasonable for the PSROs to ask the hospitals to pay. The situation was not clarified by the PSRO statute in any way, as §1168 says nothing about the way in which allocated funds should be distributed, and §1155(e), which encourages PSROs to delegate review authority, does not require hospitals to seek it.

Nor could it be said that the statute, in its silence, was relying on a historical pattern which would tend to indicate that payment should come from a single source. Where hospitals had been doing utilization review, such review had been paid for by Medicare, Medicaid, and Blue Cross or other insurers as part of the hospitals' basic day rate; it had been considered a "reasonable, ordinary, and necessary" expense of providing hospital care. However, in those areas where a Foundation for Medical Care was doing utilization review for Medicaid, the foundation was, more frequently than not, paid directly by the Medicaid state agency.[46] The funding sources and routes (to the review group, to the hospitals) varied widely.

As soon as the problem became apparent, various solutions were proposed to HEW. One, which had the virtue of simplicity, was that the PSRO program should pay for all review, reimbursing delegated hospitals (so long as their costs did not exceed some fixed ceiling) and paying the PSROs for nondelegated review and all management activities. This proposal had the disadvantage that it would make the PSRO program a highly visible item in HEW's annual budget. It is not at all clear that mandated review costs can be held below 1% of total health expenditures unless the number of cases reviewed is cut drastically;[47] and one tenth of one percent of the GNP is a lot to pay for a program which has few tangible or visible results.

Under other proposals, Medicare and Medicaid funds would pay for the reasonable and ordinary costs of doing some or all review, and a direct PSRO allocation would pay for the remaining costs of reviewing care and running the PSRO program. Under one such proposal, Medicare and Medicaid funds would have been given only to hospitals doing review, and the PSROs would have been paid out of the program allocations for doing the rest. This would have had the disadvantage of creating an incentive in favor of the PSROs' delegating, even to hospitals not capable of doing an adequate job, and would probably have tended to subvert the program.

As a result, the OPSR and BQA favored an alternative proposal under which Medicare and Medicaid funds would be given for review whether the hospital was delegated or not. Therefore, if a PSRO were doing review for a nondelegated hospital, that proportion of the PSRO's costs which were directly allocatable to inhospital review would be reimbursed out of Title XVIII and XIX funds, with the PSRO either being paid directly by SSA/SRS or being reimbursed by the hospital. Although this would probably be consistent with the language of §1168, the executive branch of the federal government chose to read that section to mean that total multiple-source funding could not exceed the direct authorization made by Congress in the line-item budget. In other words, if the Congressional instruction were to give the PSRO program $37,000,000, the executive branch would have the option of raising the entire amount from general revenues allocated to HEW or going into Medicare or Medicaid trust funds for some or all of the $37,000,000. The OPSR, of course, would have preferred an interpretation that would have read Congressional appropriations as a limit only on §1168(c) ("funds appropriated . . . "), and permitted HEW to apply additional money from the trust funds under an automatic authority granted by §1168(a) and (b).

In any case, it developed that no matter which of the above alternatives was chosen, all were at that time legally impossible. The Social Security Act [48] has been interpreted as prohibiting the expenditure of Medicaid funds for any hospital function which is not equally available to nonfederally supported patients. This brought HEW to an impasse, because low program funding prevented most PSROs from developing review plans of sufficient sensitivity to convince private third-party payors to contract with the PSROs to do review for them. As a result, an appeal was made to Congress, which responded by enacting an amendment to Section 1815 of the Social Security Act:

> Payment under this title for utilization review activities provided by a [PSRO] pursuant to an arrangement or deemed arrangement with the hospital under Section 1861(w)(2) shall be calculated without any requirement that the reasonable cost of such activities be apportioned among the patients of such hospital, if any, to whom such activities were not applicable.

The way has thus been cleared for Medicare/Medicaid funding of review activities, whether the review is conducted by the hospital or by the PSRO, so long as the PSRO law is complied with.

Interaction with Medicare and Medicaid

The problems of reimbursement and program funding are not the only ones which arise from the interaction of Title XI(B) (PSRO) with

Titles XVIII (Medicare) and XIX (Medicaid) of the Social Security Act.[49] Utilization Review, a major component of PSRO review, is, and has been, required under both Medicare and Medicaid. One of the more persistent difficulties in the PSRO program has been the problem of the phaseover and/or duplication of activities between the two older programs and PSRO.

The PSRO statute appears clear: No matter what UR programs had existed in the past in a given geographical area, the UR decisions of an operational PSRO (and, by extension, any of its delegated hospital committees) are to be binding on the Medicare and Medicaid programs in that area (§§1164, 1153). In addition, §1152(e) permits HEW to declare that a given conditional PSRO's UR decisions will also be binding. It was Congress's stated intent that PSRO review replace previous UR programs:

> ... the committee believes that the critically important utilization review process must be restructured and made more effective through substantially increased professional participation.[50]

The argument can be made that until HEW is willing to certify a given review process, either by granting full operational status or by specially finding that the conditional PSRO has the ability to do UR satisfactorily, the old programs should be maintained. Even if the statute and legislative history had not said so explicitly, common sense would dictate the same result. An operational cost-control program, even one as flawed as the Senate Finance Committee believed prior UR to be,[51] should not be scrapped until something as good or better can be substituted. In practice, however, this has meant that programs supported by the SSA (Medicare) and SRS (Medicaid) have been allowed to maintain their momentum while PSRO review procedures are slowly hammered out. It is possible that if UR had been stopped to make way for PSRO review, the PSROs would have been forced to come up to speed, at least on concurrent UR, well within the original two-year statutory deadline.

There is another, somewhat more subtle problem: the longer the phaseover is delayed (whether because of PSROs' failure to meet operational requirements or because of HEW's failure to establish them), the more likely it is that PSROs' ultimate UR processes will have to resemble those which have already been established by Medicare and Medicaid. As long as the two payor programs are willing to shape their regulations to meet the PSRO program's eventual needs, this will not be a problem; but it is possible, and perhaps even likely, that provider pressure, primarily in the form of litigation, will force the SSA and SRS to draft UR regulations which are in fact less rigorous than—if not overtly in conflict with—UR programs which would be possible and even desirable under PSRO.[52] By the time the PSRO regulations become available, hospitals may feel locked into the Medicare/Medicaid review process; they may, in fact, regard the need to change their data-collection or care-evaluation methods as a serious disincentive to application for delegated status. This would tend to complicate the PSRO's manpower problems at both the review-coordinator and physician-reviewer levels.

There is another phaseover problem: many state Medicaid agencies have invested time, money, effort, and their political reputations into the development of UR systems.[53] If PSRO review is less effective than the states' systems at containing Medicaid costs, even after the PSROs have become fully operational, it would be financially—and therefore politically—unwise to switch from the more effective state system to the less effective subregional PSRO program. If, on the other hand, PSRO review is more effective at containing Medicaid costs than are the state-developed programs, that would demonstrate that the very physicians and hospitals who have the most to lose by effective implementation can in fact do a better job than can the various state health bureaucrats. The political repercussions of such a demonstration are not hard to imagine.

As far as the PSRO program is concerned, therefore, the longer full operational implementation is delayed, the more likely it is that political arguments will be found to keep it from ever being implemented. While the fight between the vested interests at SSA/SRS and the BQA can be refereed by the Secretary of HEW, until §1164 becomes active no one in the federal program can effectively tell the states how to spend their own Medicaid funds; although HEW can, of course, restrict the use to which federal Medicaid funds are devoted, and even decrease the federal contribution if a state Medicaid agency is too recalcitrant. The result is that some states have threatened to maintain duplicate UR programs until forced (by §1164) to dismantle them. However politically satisfactory such a solution might be to those involved, maintenance of duplicate systems to review the same patients for the same reasons in the same way is financially wasteful. It ought not be encouraged by anyone within HEW or the medical professions.

THE MANUALS AND TRANSMITTALS

How does a government agency run a program without issuing regulations? In the case of the PSRO program, the answer is clear: it issues nonbinding "guidelines" which it then makes binding through the use of the contracts process. So far, the "guidelines" have appeared in two forms: manuals and transmittals.

Since March 15, 1974, when the Office of Professional Standards Review (OPSR) in HEW issued the first seven chapters of the *PSRO Program Manual*, there have been two more manuals (the *PSRO Management Information System Manual*, or *PMIS Manual*; and the *PSRO Contract Management Manual*, or *CCM*), some additional chapters of the *Program Manual*, and 36 transmittal letters.[54] The manuals and transmittals contain HEW's detailed instructions to PSROs on everything from methods of organizing to data collection to budget accounting; or, in other words, the actual operating requirements of the PSRO program.

And yet, technically, neither the manuals nor the transmittal letters contain regulations, as that term is understood by lawyers and defined by federal law. Does it make any difference?

Until early 1976, the answer appeared to be "no." Because HEW's contracts with the PSROs made the guidelines as binding as regulations, the guidelines were, in fact, largely obeyed, and the PSRO program moved forward at the pace set for it by HEW. Nevertheless, it was no secret that some PSROs resented "regulation by contract,"[55] although they appear to have been unwilling, or felt unable, to attack it. In May 1976, their ranks were joined by the states of Massachusetts, Hawaii, Kentucky, and Ohio, which were tired of waiting for the regulations on confidentiality to appear and sued HEW to compel the regulation-writing process to begin. Massachusetts' Attorney General instituted the suit and solicited other states' participation at the request of the state's assistant attorney general in charge of consumer protection. Their concern may have been triggered by a policy statement on confidentiality from the Bay State PSRO (Massachusetts' largest) in which, relying on Transmittal 16, Bay State had severely restricted consumers' access to information supplied to and generated by the PSRO. The lawsuit asked that HEW be forced to follow the procedures established by the federal Administrative Procedures Act in establishing regulations on the confidentiality of PSRO data, and that it be forced to do so immediately.

Should the plaintiffs win? The answer is "yes." [56]

The arguments against HEW's policy of control by contract rest on two statutory bases: 5 USC 552 and 553, part of the Administrative Procedures Act, and §§1152(d), 1155(a)(3), 1155(b), 1155(f)(1)(A), 1156(b), 1156(d)(1)(A), 1158(a), 1160(b)(2), 1162(c), 1162(e)(2), 1165, and 1166(a) of the Social Security Act, all parts of the PSRO law. As the foregoing list indicates, there are twelve places in the PSRO law where

HEW has been explicitly instructed by Congress that if it wishes to take action it must first promulgate regulations; only on the question of hospital delegation is HEW given the option of avoiding the regulatory process. Of particular interest to those who resent control by guidelines pursuant to contract is §1155(f)(1)(A), which reads, in pertinent part:

> An agreement entered into... between the Secretary [of HEW] and any [PSRO] shall provide that such organization will—(A) perform such duties... and comply with such other requirements as may be required by this [law] or under regulations of the Secretary promulgated to carry out the provisions of this [law]; and (B) collect such data... and maintain such records in such form as the Secretary may require....

One notes immediately that the statute appears to prohibit HEW from requiring a PSRO to meet any requirements outside of the statute itself unless such requirements assume the form of promulgated regulations, except, possibly, in the area of data collection. It is safe to presume that where Congress says "regulations... promulgated" it is referring to 5 USC 552 and 553.

Section 552 (§3 of the APA) requires all federal agencies to publish, in the *Federal Register,*

> substantive rules adopted as authorized by law and... interpretations adopted by the agency for public guidance, except rules addressed to and served on named persons in accordance with law.

The rule applies to all cases other than those involving "secrecy in the public interest" or "internal management of an agency." Section 553 (§4 of the APA) requires publication of "notice[s] of proposed rule making," including the text of the proposed rule, citation of the agency's legal authority for the making of the rule, and "a statement of the time, place, and nature of public rule making proceedings," if any are to be held. Proposed rules, like actual rules, need not be published if they are served on named persons, or involve national security or internal agency management; there are some additional exceptions which are not relevant to the PSRO program. It is §553 which provides that there must be a minimum of 30 days between publications of proposed and final rules in most cases.

The basic purpose of the Administrative Procedures Act is to give those people who are or will be affected by agencies' rules a chance to influence those rules, or at least see what they are, during at least a short period prior to their imposition, as well as during the time they are in force. Courts are expected to construe exceptions to the act's procedures narrowly, and in general they do.[57] As long as HEW continues to try to circumvent the act, its ability to control the PSRO program is vulnerable to attack.

As for the specific attack being mounted by the four states on behalf of consumer access to PSRO data, HEW's only defenses are likely to be those listed in §553 itself: that confidentiality of data is either a matter of purely internal agency management (unlikely, especially if PSROs are held to be independent corporations), or a general statement of policy (again unlikely, especially if the PSROs are instructed to institute or maintain specific procedures), or that all persons affected by the rules "have actual notice" through the manuals and/or transmittals (acceptable only if the court is willing to grant the argument that data confidentiality does not affect patients or nonmember practitioners). To some extent, all these defenses, however weak, are further vitiated by §1166(a) of the PSRO law, which provides that acquired data "shall not be disclosed...except...[as] necessary to carry out the purposes of [the statute] or...in such cases...as the Secretary shall *by regulations* provide..." (italics added).

In a very real sense, however, the plight of the PSROs is more basic than that of the consumers' advocates who are objecting to HEW's failure to go through a public rule-development process. The PSROs' problem is that HEW's refusal goes beyond public rule-making to private rule-making, so that the PSROs are denied the rights apparently promised by §1155(f)(1)(A) and §552, and, perhaps more to the point, cannot refer to published regulations in defense of their contract-abiding actions when challenged by any outsider who claims to be aggrieved by something they have done. In at least one case, the absence of published regulations would have been extremely material, if not actually dispositive, in a lawsuit which was brought against a PSRO; and the absence of those regulations, which the PSRO might have used in defending its position, may have been a factor in the settlement of the case before trial.[58]

While it is understandable that the Deputy Assistant Secretary for Quality Assurance (DASQA, which replaced the old OPSR) and the Bureau of Quality Assurance (BQA) in HEW, understaffed as they are, might wish to forgo the troublesome and time-consuming process of complying with Administrative Procedures Act rule-making processes, such avoidance becomes increasingly risky as the PSRO program moves from organizational to operational phases. While it might be successfully argued that Transmittal 5, on the expenditure of federal funds for travel, has been "addressed to and served on"[59] all persons affected, it is considerably harder to prove that the PSRO personnel who are the sole recipients of the more recent transmittals, (such as #24, on coordination with state Medicaid agencies, or #27, on the financing of delegated review), are the only persons affected by the decisions contained therein. And if the statutory defenses cannot be made, HEW is violating federal law.

All that having been said, what of the transmittals and manuals themselves? At the moment, legally unreliable though they may be, they are the only "law" available other than the statute and three or four sets of final regulations (e.g., on area designation, notice, and polling; or on hearings and appeals at the federal level). Of the 36 transmittals issued, seven (the largest number on a single subject) have dealt with data—paperwork, to the cynic—; five have dealt with various aspects of the PSRO-UR interface; four have covered delegation of review authority to hospitals; and the rest have been concerned with such subjects as continuing education, coordination with state Medicaid agencies, contract management and subcontracting, and tax exemptions. A table of the published transmittals appears in Appendix E.

The only transmittals likely to be of long-term interest are those on the delegation of review authority to hospitals, as the PSRO statute will not force HEW to produce regulations in that area unless it tries to bind PSROs to a specific delegation process and set of criteria by contract. The *PSRO Program Manual* and Transmittals 11, 15, 27 and 34 do, respectively, establish a generalized delegation process (Manual §§710 and 720, and Transmittal 11, which actually disagree slightly on minor points), a framework within which reimbursement can be arranged (Transmittals 27 and 34), and a procedure for reconsidering the decisions made pursuant to Transmittal 11 (Transmittal 15); yet it cannot be said that any of these guidelines are so precise or restrictive that they would be a significant constraint on any affected PSRO or other party. Even the most specific of the group, #11, merely establishes a six-step process, from initial contact to final decision, which, if followed, would enable the PSRO and hospitals to reach agreement simultaneously while providing HEW with the documentation it needs as a basis for any rational decision to approve or deny the PSRO's delegations should the matter reach appeal. To the extent that the HEW-PSRO contracts require PSROs to use this process, of course, the transmittals should be replaced by regulations. As it appears, however, that more necessary regulations have yet to be written, one can understand why no PSRO has tried to force the issue. Half a loaf may well be better than none, and to invalidate the guidelines is not to write their replacement.

An index to the *Program Manual* and transmittals can be found in Appendix D.

LEGAL CONCERNS

This chapter has been designed to show how the PSRO law—statute and regulations—was designed by Congress and shaped by HEW, and to demonstrate how and where PSRO operations will resemble and differ from the UR and medical audit processes from which the federal concept was derived. In so doing, it has occasionally been useful to mention briefly some of the practical or political pressures which have helped shape the PSRO program. But is should be obvious that such discussion has so far been minimal and inadequate. What a law says on paper is only the beginning. How the law is applied—and, ultimately, whether it stands or falls—depends not only on how well it was drafted but on how desperately those who are affected by it need to alter or abolish it. And the PSRO law, which has received less public attention than most Medicare and Medicaid laws, has created nothing but controversy within the medical and other health care professions. Are the worries justified? Are the reassurances based on facts? The next chapters will be concerned with what is at stake (money, professional autonomy, the quality of medical care, scientific progress) and with some of the legal weapons available to those who wish to attack the program and those who would defend it. The impact of PSROs on malpractice, malpractice litigation, licensure, confidentiality, and privacy will be considered as will the impact of malpractice costs and laws, hospital staff law, the laws dealing with defamation (libel and slander) and testimonial privilege, and the Constitution of the United States on PSROs.

NOTES

1. §1151, 42 USC 1320c. A table of cross-citations to the U.S. Code is appended. Hereinafter, textual citations will be limited to Social Security Act section numbers; footnote citations will include both.

2. S. Rept. No. 92-1230, p. 254. [hereinafter Fin. Comm. Rept.]

3. For example, the no-crossing-of-state-boundaries rule. See, in general, B. Decker and P. Bonner, *PSRO: Organization for Regional Peer Review* (1973).

4. For example, the Texas Medical Association's willingness to go to court over the question of state-level control of the PSRO program.

5. Legislative history is to be used by courts only when the statute itself fails to provide a clear meaning.

6. Fin. Comm. Rept. 258, 259.

7. *PSRO Program Manual.*

8. Texas Medical Association v. Mathews, 408 F. Supp. 303 (1976).

9. S. Rept. No. 94-549, p. 10.

10. B. Mackey, "Results of PSRO Balloting," *PSRO Update* n. 25 (1976). See also 41 FR 50347—50352, reporting, *inter alia*, the results of the balloting in Louisiana. The general procedures for statewide redesignation can be found at 42 CFR 101.2a, first promulgated in 41 CFR 33436—33437 (August 9, 1976).

11. PL 94-182, §108(b)(1).

12. §1152(b)(2), 42 USC 1320c-1(b)(2).

13. §1154(a), 42 USC 1320c-3(a).

14. *Id.*

15. §1154(b), 42 USC 1320c–3(b).

16. *Id.*

17. This requirement has been more honored in the breach than in the observance. The statute itself does not explicitly command HEW to terminate funding, but if a PSRO remains unqualified at the end of its 24-month statutory maximum trial period, what alternative does HEW have? The argument can be made that on this question the statute was badly drafted, as the Finance Committee's original report implied that the consequence of nonqualification would be that there would be no waiver of other review regulations (Fin. Comm. Rept. at 264), but did not contemplate a funding cutoff.

18. There are fewer PSROs than PSRO areas, and, in fact, there has rarely been competition for review authority within any given designated area; the real competition has been for the limited federal funds.

19. §1152(b), 42 USC 1320c-1(b): "the term 'qualified organization' means . . . a nonprofit professional association. . . ."

20. See PSRO Transmittal No. 6.

21. 39 FR 16202, 42 CFR 101(B). A modification was made in 1976 (41 FR 17865, amending 42 CFR 101.100 and 101.103) to conform to the changes mandated by P.L. 94-182, §108 (§1152(c) and 1152(f)). See also 41 FR 29995.

22. §1155(a)(1)(c), 42 USC 1320c-4(a)(1)(c). But see proposed rules for PSRO review in 42 FR 4620, 4628—4629.

23. Am. Med. Assn. v. Weinberger, 522 F.2d 921 (1975).

24. Retrospective review is permitted by §1155(b), 42 USC 1320c-4(b).

25. Fin. Comm. Rept. at 257.

26. Id.

27. HEW's use of "standard," as was remarked in chapter 1, can be ambiguous. In general, the word must be interpreted as "acceptable deviation from the norm" whenever it occurs in most pre-1977 HEW communications. It is not at all clear that Congress intended the word's meaning in the statute to be limited in that manner. HEW appears to have modified its definition recently to permit physicians' judgments in the standards-setting process: see the proposed rules at 42 FR 4627 (January 25, 1977).

28. Unless the "professional" being referred to is a professional statistician. A program which pays only for normative care can be run by a computer; a program which relies on profile review to develop "standards" need not waste physicians' time in making judgments.

29. HEW appears to agree. See proposed rule 42 CFR 101.713(c) at 42 FR 4631.

30. Frank A. Howard Mem. Hosp. v. Redwood Coast PSRO, Cal. Super. Ct. #36278 Mendaceno Co. (1975).

31. Fin. Comm. Rept. at 265.

32. HEW's proposed regulations say "shall." Proposed 42 CFR 101.712(a) at 42 FR 4631.

33. A simple example: miscoding can easily lead to errors in the assignment of length-of-stay review dates, with obvious consequences.

34. Whether the law will actually be obeyed is, at the present time, open to question.

35. 41 FR 7877-7879.

36. §1166(b), 42 USC 1320c-15(b).

37. This is obviously a simplistic example. The causes of nonstandard physician behavior vary widely, and in some cases can result from a combination of patient-generated and physician-generated difficulties. Furthermore, reviewers' judgments vary; what one reviewer regards as suboptimal another may see as perfectly acceptable. Although MCEs may eventually provide control for this sort of reviewer variation, concurrent UR may not.

38. Information derived from private conversations. It is probable, however, that this phenomenon will occur primarily during the earliest periods of PSRO operation; after that, the physicians who are willing to correct themselves will probably have done so, and only the more intransigent will be left.

39. §1156, 42 USC 1320c-5.

40. See §1155(a), 42 USC 1320c-4(a).

41. Some PSRO personnel, at least in private conversation, admit that education in itself is not very effective in improving care. For education to work, the practitioner must believe he needs help; sometimes a forceful demonstration (e.g., by the consultant) is necessary to convince the practitioner of his need. (See subsection on Consultation).

42. Indirect impairment is a very real possibility, because many hospitals require specialty certification as a precondition for the granting of practice privileges in certain fields, particularly advanced surgery. If and when a physician in such a hospital has his certification revoked, the hospital has the power either to revoke or to fail to renew his practice privileges.

43. It should also be remembered by the PSRO that the state licensure agency can, in certain instances, subpoena the physician profiles, which raises a pertinent legal issue: if the agency merely asks, the PSRO may be within its rights in refusing to supply the profile; if the agency has subpoena power and exercises it validly, the PSRO may have no choice but to submit the profile to the state agency. Such release, however, may be prohibited if the physician does not authorize it, if the ultimate HEW regulations resemble the draft guidelines published to date. If a report is made to a state medical society which has disciplinary powers, of course, there could be a real possibility of immediate and direct curtailment of the physician's professional activities.

44. Fin. Comm. Rept. at 266.

45. It cannot be said that it was Congress's intent to starve the program, but rather that the PSRO program got caught in the Congressional backlash of the late Nixon years. The fiscal 1974 PSRO appropriation was $32,850,000 (of which $13,244,132 was awarded to 11 conditional PSROs; $5,520,694 to 91 planning PSROs; $2,085,493 to 13 state Support Centers; and the remainder stayed within HEW). By the time funds ran out, review programs had actually been started by fewer than 11 PSROs. Cost savings attributable to PSRO, if any existed, were undocumented. When HEW asked Congress for a fiscal 1975 appropriation of $57,000,000 for the program, the House responded by marking up an allocation of

$36,208,000, which the Senate agreed to. As a result, contract awards for the second year of program operations included $20,445,601 to conditional PSROs and $5,813,926 to planning PSROs. Funding has been less of a constraint since then: in the five quarters of fiscal 1976, total appropriations were $59,622,000 ($45,050,383 conditional; $2,459,404 planning); in fiscal 1977, $61,125,000, of which an estimated $41,860,000 has gone to approximately 120 conditionals and an estimated $10,375,000 to planning PSROs in the remaining areas; additionally, an estimated $41,000,000 in Medicare Trust Funds will be used to pay for review in all delegated and nondelegated hospitals.

46. In some cases this resulted in what was essentially a double billing of UR costs to Medicaid and concomitant underpayment by Medicare and the private insurers. For example, in Massachusetts, hospitals which had UR committees and the necessary administrative backup had been aggregating utilization review costs, dividing the aggregate by the number of patient days, and charging the payors per day accordingly. The state's Medicaid monitoring program (CHAMP), run by Medicaid and a local medical care foundation, provided its own administrative backup to the hospital's UR committees, so that to the extent that Medicaid paid for hospital administrative backup in UR, it paid twice. Medicare and the others, of course, ended up paying less than their fair share.

47. There is some evidence that, at present, UR costs approximately one percent of reviewed (institutional) care. For example, in the Boston area in 1975–76, UR cost approximately $1.25 per patient per day, and the average day's stay in an acute care bed cost $125.00. While ancillary and ambulatory care adds significantly to patients' total cost, such care is not reviewed. When it is, review costs might again reach one percent or more of the total. When one considers predictions that health costs may constitute ten percent of the GNP before becoming somewhat stabilized, 1/10% of the GNP would not be an outrageous guess for total review costs, were it not also probable that either Congress or HEW will move to cut costs before they reach that level.

48. *Medicare Hospital Manual* (HIM 10) §290.

49. Title V (Maternal & Child Health) is not included in this discussion because it is not subject to PSROs except for data-gathering purposes; §1158(a), 42 USC 1320c-7(a), prohibits PSROs from making reimbursement decisions for Title V cases.

50. Fin. Comm. Rept. at 256.

51. Id., at 255.

52. See Chapter 4 and the discussion of §1152(a)(2), 42 USC 1320c-1(a)(2), earlier in this chapter. It should also be noted that §1903(g)(1)(c) has been read as prohibiting "universal" UR.

53. See Chapter 1.

54. As of July 1, 1976.

55. D. Willett, "PSRO Today: A Lawyer's Assessment," 292 *New England J. Med.*, pp. 340, 341: "Reliance on the contracting process to establish and regulate PSROs is inappropriate for several reasons. In the first place . . . the contracting process . . . is not a public process. . . . The concerned public . . . will have difficulty in learning about or influencing contractual provisions before adoption. . . . further . . . the parties to the process hardly stand in parity. . . ."

56. As of July 1, 1976, the case had not yet been argued, and in late 1976 HEW moved to moot the suit by beginning the rule-making process with the issuance of interim final regulations on data disclosure (42 CFR 101.1701 and 101.1702). It should be noted that, in addition to the complaint discussed in the text, the plaintiffs hoped to compel HEW to

hold hearings. Success on this count is considerably less likely, as the matter is entirely discretionary with HEW.

57. The only major exception to this requirement (aside from the exceptions listed in 5 USC 553 itself) is one which originally grew out of the case law: when an agency decides cases that have been brought to a hearing before it, it may create law/regulation by precedent, just as the judiciary creates law by precedent. As a result, rule-making through adjudication is recognized in the same way as rule-making through the Administrative Procedures Act regulatory process.

58. 5 USC 552(b)(3).

59. Frank A. Howard Mem. Hosp. v. Redwood Coast PSRO, supra, note 30.

Chapter 3

Providers' Concerns about the PSRO Program

Congressional concerns about the PSRO program can be said to be relatively straightforward: Can PSROs cut Medicare/Medicaid costs without lowering quality? Will the PSRO program cost more than it saves? The same, however, cannot be said for the concerns of those who are most directly affected by the program: hospitals, nursing homes, physicians, nurses, and other health care personnel. The argument can be made that the ultimate effect—and effectiveness—of the PSRO program will depend on the way providers' problems are solved and conflicts resolved.

Discussions of the PSRO program have tended, perhaps properly, to mingle cost- and quality-related issues. And yet, while most authors and Senate witnesses generally agree that medical costs and health quality may be closely intertwined, the discussion has been somewhat hampered by a fact which many participants frankly admit: the "cost-quality tradeoff" is not easily quantifiable. Other confusions in the debate over PSRO, however, may be ripe for clarification. Opposition to the PSRO program by some provider organizations[1] has been intensive and emotional; debate has frequently been characterized by exaggeration, and occasionally by outright misrepresentation of fact.[2] By far the largest portion of the debate, however, centers not on fact but on projections of future developments with those who favor the program generally predicting that HEW will read its mandate narrowly, and those who dislike the program predicting that HEW will take over the medical and/or hospital profession. Additionally, all sides have tended to portray themselves as struggling underdogs and their opponents as overbearing tyrants. Neither of these views is strictly true. The debate's being emotional may be the result of the program's having been instituted before adequate research was done to determine its effects. In

59

the absence of known facts, the participants understandably are projecting their fears and hopes onto a program which remains, more than two years after its inception, not yet fully implemented.

Nevertheless, some facts are known or at least knowable. Existing utilization review programs resemble some aspects of PSRO-mandated review enough for observers to draw some probably valid conclusions.

COSTS

An obvious fact about the PSRO program is that it will be expensive. Peer review costs money. And PSRO review may become more costly than any previous review program because PSROs have a broad scope of operations, potentially higher administrative costs, and are tied to at least one review methodology (concurrent periodic recertification) whose long-term cost/benefit ratio has not yet been proved favorable. Any analysis of PSRO costs must consider the following:

Salaries and Overheads. As in many pre-PSRO review programs, review coordinators (nurse reviewers) will almost inevitably be salaried workers. Private peer review organizations have tended to find that review coordinators' salaries must be competitive with the salaries of similarly trained nurses in the organization's geographical area. This is because review coordinators must be specially talented (able to communicate well with physicians, nurses, etc.) and specially trained; so that, in a competitive market, available personnel are able to command a higher salary than they might otherwise, considering the nonfinancial compensations of the review coordinators' job, which include regular hours, freedom from weekend work, and, for many coordinators, increased professional status and responsibility.

Where PSRO differs from most earlier review programs is in the additional professional fees PSROs apparently have to pay to encourage physicians to serve as advisors and committee members. Three reasons for this additional "salary" cost have been suggested. The first is simply that the money is available; many earlier programs were funded by the physicians themselves, and taking a fee would have been robbing Peter to pay Paul. Second, PSRO participation promises to be more time-consuming than participation in other programs. PSROs must monitor quality as well as cost, and the law demands that review criteria in most cases be explicit[3] and subject to periodic re-evaluation and possible modification.[4] Therefore, service on criteria-setting and review committees has an enormous potential for consuming more time than participating physicians can afford to spare from their practices.[5] Third, the program does not possess the loyalty and commitment of a significant portion of the country's physicians. Although many appear to be willing to give the program a chance,[6] few are so committed to it that they are willing to serve without some kind of compensation. If PSRO review proves to be useful to the medical profession, it is possible that future compensation might be nonfinancial (e.g., increased prestige as a result of participation). Until then, however, money seems to be a good, if not the best, incentive. It should be noted that if physicians insist that they will not accept payment at a level lower than professional earnings for comparable periods of time, PSROs' professional fees could be a substantial cost. At one time, HEW tried to limit such reimbursement to a maximum of $35 per hour.[7]

Whether the reviewing organization is a PSRO, a foundation, or a hospital, it must expect to have to pay management and administrative salaries, buy office equipment and supplies, lease telephones and office space, purchase meals, travel, and, in general, incur all those routine overheads normally associated with any business enterprise. When the reviewing organization is a PSRO or delegated hospital rather than a private program, however, these overhead costs will inevitably be increased by the need to meet federal reporting requirements.

Actually, when the question of paperwork arises, the PSRO program is caught on the horns of a dilemma. It would ultimately be cheaper for all PSROs to collect data in a single format, whether on paper or tape, use a single coding system, and simply forward a copy of their papers or computer tapes to HEW during that agency's legally required[8] periodic evaluations of PSROs' performance. HEW could get the medical and financial information it needed without the PSROs' having to convert or translate their data. The trouble with such a system is that the ultimate savings could be purchased only by an enormous and possibly prohibitive initial expenditure of time and money. This is because many of the medical organizations which received early conditional designation had been doing review for varying periods of time with computer systems, data abstracts, and coding terminology that they considered sufficiently accurate and financially acceptable. That the systems were not mutually compatible was of little importance to the new PSROs, and HEW, following Congressional suggestions,[9] agreed that making the program operational (as the statute defines operational) was to take precedence over making it easy to administer in the long run. As a result, the systems are firmly entrenched, and the job of conversion, expensive at the outset, has worsened. Such conversion will become increasingly costly as more and more PSROs become dependent on new data-processing systems. HEW therefore has apparently decided not to insist on nation-wide uniformity of data-processing systems, efficient as that would be, but rather demands special periodic reports from each PSRO.[10] These special reports, necessary though they are, constitute a definite additional overhead cost for any PSRO; and the more reports HEW needs, the higher the cost.

Data Processing. HEW reports aside, PSROs, like other peer review groups, will largely be information-processing organizations. In those PSROs or hospitals which rely to any extent on automated data processing, the cost of computer time, if not the computers themselves, will be a major budget item. Additionally, a certain number of personnel (typists and/or keypunchers, maintenance workers, programmers, and management personnel) will be needed to see that the data are properly fed into the computers, that the hardware (machines) and software (programs) work properly, and that the resulting data will be produced on schedule and in a usable format. If the PSRO or hospital has its own computer, it will pay for these people directly; if, as seems likely to be the usual case, it buys time from a data processor, the data processing personnel salaries will be part of the total cost package presented by the processor to the PSRO or hospital.

The basic costs of PSRO data processing (personnel and paper if nonautomated; personnel, paper, and computer system if automated) are unavoidable, given that HEW will demand certain minimum data from every PSRO. (See, for example, PSRO transmittal letters 9, 20, 25, 26, and 28, or the PMIS Manual.) Inter-PSRO cost differences are likely to be most directly related to regional salary differences and less directly related to the complexity of basic data-gathering as long as each PSRO confines itself to meeting minimal federal requirements.[11] If, however, some PSROs wish to extend their range, for example, into ambulatory review, increased program complexity and computer storage capacity could significantly increase costs.

Other significant variables in data processing costs will be the degree of access to the data which the PSRO or hospital permits and the degree of data identifiability which it maintains. These are not inversely related. A PSRO or hospital performing non-PSRO review may decide to provide strictly limited access (e.g., no researchers, no nonreview usage) and a high degree of nonidentifiability (reviewed individuals are identified in the system only by a hospital- or PSRO-generated number), wide access (researchers and consumers permitted to look routinely at non-identifiable data) and medium identifiability (patients and physicians identified by Social Security number), moderate access and easy identifiability (listing by name), or any combination of access and identifiability. The PSRO's or hospital's choice will have cost implications because, in general, the more elaborate the security system, in the computer or in the office, the more expensive. A computer system without elaborate checks of passwords or its own identifier for each patient is cheaper than a system that has such safeguards. Confidentiality, while desirable, has its price.

Quality Monitoring. If PSROs meet their legal mandate to monitor the quality of, as well as the necessity for, medical care provided under the Medicare and Medicaid programs, the PSRO program could become as heavily involved in monitoring quality as the Medicare and Medicaid programs are presently involved in UR. While the costs of UR are largely known, the costs of monitoring quality, which are particularly dependent on the methodology used, cannot be reliably assessed at this time. It is probable, however, that quality-monitoring costs will be higher than UR costs for any given group of patients. This is because the criteria-development process for quality review is considerably more complex than the same process for UR. In fact, it is possible to think of UR as a type of review for which most of the necessary criteria-development work has already been performed.[12] For quality review, on the other hand, the criteria-establishment policy is comparatively complex and by no means standardized. A significantly larger number of people, most of whom will be required to hold medical degrees, will be involved in developing and reviewing both process and outcome criteria. And because the criteria-developers' decisions can have ethical and legal implications (unlike the decision to set a UR length-of-stay checkpoint at day x rather than day y), the criteria-setting process can be expected to be more protracted, and therefore more expensive, than if a merely academic review system were being devised.

In some cases, the higher costs of criteria development for quality review can be wholly or partially offset by potentially lower costs for the quality review itself. Chart-abstracting for the simplest types of quality review can be performed at a single sitting, and if the quality review is retrospective rather than concurrent, the costs should be reduced even further. If, however, the quality-review methodology chosen by the PSRO or other peer review group is relatively complex, or if the organization's review criteria are being evaluated (or reevaluated) along with the physicians' records, the review process will demand relatively large amounts of physicians' and other professionals' time, and there will be a corresponding increase in cost.

It is probably fair to say that the only certain way to limit the cost of quality review is to limit the number of patients reviewed. If full-scale quality review is universal, patients' and physicians' demands for ever-more-careful discrimination between the avoidable and the unavoidable bad result, between acceptable deviant practice and malpractice, are likely to push the review system to cost levels beyond those the country can afford. If, on the other hand, quality review involves a comparatively miniscule number of patients' charts, the reviews themselves could be made rather sophisticated without the cost of review outrunning the program's budget.

The inevitability of high program costs has not gone unnoticed. For example, in testimony before the Health Subcommittee of the Senate Finance Committee on May 9, 1974, Dr. James Stewart of the Louisiana State Medical Society asked the Senate to consider permitting "substantially less than full scale implementation"[13] for reasons which included the following:

> Our estimates suggest that fully operational [PSROs] will cost in excess of $100 million per year, and this does not include the various support and advisory organizations that may be formed. Now, this is more than $100 million per year in added administrative costs of Federal health programs; not one cent would go to health care itself. The question of recovery of some or all of this cost by bringing about curtailment of services under this program is a theory lacking in substantive proof.[14]

While some costs, such as universal preadmission screening or duplication of review systems by state Medicaid agencies, are avoidable, or at least could be minimized by timely intervention by HEW, the concern that the PSRO program itself not cost more than its potential savings has become increasingly worrisome to provider groups and government personnel. Concern has increased as the realization has grown that cost savings generated by review programs (which will be discussed in the next section) cannot be expected to continue to outrun direct-cost increases which appear inevitable at this time.[15] It also appears that doubts about the ultimate cost-effectiveness of PSROs and PSRO-type review programs are a factor in physician and hospital opposition, although obviously not as important a factor as the fear of direct financial loss.

From the institutional point of view, it would be preferable to have the direct costs of review borne by the PSRO or outside private peer review organization. This would neither increase nor decrease the hospital's net revenue. The worst alternative would be for the hospital to have to pay for review without receiving any reimbursement.

Under what circumstances would reimbursement be at less than cost? There are primarily two ways in which the hospital or other reviewed institution could lose money as a result of a financial transaction with a peer review organization, whether PSRO or private.

The hospital will suffer a financial loss if: (1) the PSRO-hospital contract locks the hospital into paying more for review than it can recover from patients and their insurers; or (2) the PSRO and hospital have contracted for review at a cost affordable by both, but which is then declared by the state's hospital-rate-setting agency not to be recoverable by the hospital. In either case, the hospital has two alternatives: back out of the contract, if possible; or hide review costs on its books, in which case patients not being reviewed may end up paying for it. Obviously, hospitals in states that have rate-setting agencies should make sure that their contracts with PSROs, including memoranda of understanding, contain clauses voiding the agreement if rate-setting agency approval cannot be obtained for any required cost increases.

An argument can be made for the claim that the payment mechanism (HEW to PSRO to delegated hospital; patient to hospital to PSRO; HEW to PSRO and patient to hospital; or whatever) is irrelevant, and that what counts, to both the institution and the PSRO or other review group, is the net amount available for financial support of the review process. As the discussion in chapter 2 indicates, this is probably a correct view, at least from the institutional perspective. If the available reimbursement covers direct costs, it should not matter to reviewers or reviewed where the money comes from. If the reimbursement is insufficient, it is obviously in the hospitals' best interest to see that HEW, or whoever funds the review program, selects a payment mechanism in which the loss falls on the reviewing organization rather than the hospital. Similarly, the PSRO would like to see the hospital bear the risk of insufficient funding. As a result, inadequate program funding is likely to lead to an impasse in PSRO-hospital negotiations at an early stage, effectively precluding any review which might have been possible.

COST IMPACTS

The Effect on Institutions

Even assuming that methods and levels of reimbursement are established which enable institutional medical providers maintain current services and costs as well as pay for review programs, institutional providers will still find themselves the reviewers' adversaries in a number of situations. Direct review costs aside, the indirect costs of peer review, whether federal or private, can fall heavily on an institution. What are these indirect costs?

Payment Denials and Cost-Shifting

Payment denial effects can range from harmless to debilitating. While a theoretically perfect hospital would never get certification denied for any patients, in the real world, of course, such no-pay decisions happen more or less frequently, and their effects can vary from moderately annoying to bankrupting. Bankruptcy, however desirable it may seem to health planners in an "overbedded" area, is unlikely except where a vigilant rate-setting agency is involved. If peer review does result in the elimination or significant reduction of unnecessary hospitalizations, hospitals which depended to any extent on revenue derived from such hospitalizations will be forced to increase charges in other areas or suffer financial loss.

Strictly speaking, this phenomenon is a cost transfer rather than a cost increase, but some commentators consider it unfortunate that the costs will be transferred to those sickest patients whose outlay is already the highest. On the other hand, there is little justification for making patients who apparently do not need hospitalization subsidize the more ill. If hospital subsidies are necessary, the argument goes, they should be paid by society as a whole rather than by patients who could be treated as safely on an outpatient or ambulatory basis. While many institutional providers might concede the justice of such an argument, their trepidation when contemplating the interim period is understandable, especially in those states where hospital-rate-setting agencies can be expected to deny or delay approval of changes in cost-allocation methods.

The type of review system chosen by the PSRO or other peer review organization will significantly influence the severity of payment-denial effects. Two examples can demonstrate this, one from utilization and one from quality review.

If the PSRO chooses a comparatively simple UR system, assigning length-of-stay checkpoints on the basis of a small number of categories (e.g., disease or reason for admission, sex, and age), hospitals which take a higher-than-average number of complicated cases will find that either their medical staffs will be forced to spend more time than they did previously documenting the medical necessity for long in-patient lengths of stay, or their number of denials will increase, or both. If the PSRO's UR system is more complex (e.g., categorizes patients by number of concurrent unrelated diseases in addition to the above three categories, or controls in some other fashion for differences in case mix) the impact will be relatively less severe.

If the PSRO's quality-monitoring system looks only at the "process" of care* rather than the outcomes of care,** the number of procedures done, although not necessarily of drugs prescribed, will inevitably increase.[16] If the hospital's patient population can pay for the mandated procedures, the hospital may actually benefit financially from the imposition of PSRO review. If the patients' or their insurers' resources are more limited, however, the hospital may suffer severely if the PSRO insists on process review. If, on the other hand, the PSRO implements outcomes-based quality review, the financial impact of such review may be significantly less serious.

It should also be noted that payment denials may fall more heavily on some types of institutions than on others no matter which review methodology is chosen. Representatives of public (city and state) institutions (federal hospitals are exempt from PSRO review), smaller community-based hospitals (especially in rural or isolated areas), teaching hospitals and specialty hospitals have all expressed serious concern.

a. *Public Acute-Care Hospitals.* Tax-supported medical facilities tend to be underfunded even in prosperous times; during depressions, declining tax revenues and increased public demand can lead to reductions in staff-to-patient ratios, failures to replace broken or overused equipment, shortages of drugs and medical supplies, and all the other problems that commonly leap to mind when the words "city hospital" are uttered. While PSRO review will identify the resulting prolonged lengths of stay and, possibly, the less successful treatment outcomes, it is not clear that appropriate remedial action will be financially possible. For the tax-supported city hospital, therefore, PSRO review means reductions in Medicaid and Medicare funding with no apparent compensatory benefit.

Unfortunately, the public hospitals' problems do not end with their own financial squeeze. If PSRO review becomes financially burdensome to surrounding private hospitals, those hospitals may attempt to reduce

---

*I.e., the criteria-setting group decides that disease x should be treated by processes a, b, and c, and drugs d and e but not f, and charts are abstracted and physicians evaluated on that basis.

**E.g., the criteria-setting group decides that treatment for disease x should cost between $1000 and $3500, result in a length of stay of between 4 and 18 days (depending on other factors), be attended by no more than 5% mortality during hospitalization, and lead to between 2 and 10 out-patient visits in the four weeks immediately following discharge.

their costs by refusing admission to, or transferring, Medicare and Medicaid patients who cannot themselves pay for care which might be "denied" by the PSRO. Those patients, whose unmet social needs traditionally lead to more-frequent-than-average denials as a result of after-care placement problems, will have nowhere to go other than to the already struggling public hospitals, thus making a bad situation worse.

b. *Small Hospitals.* PSRO review worries small rural hospitals for the same reason that it worries big urban hospitals: the rural hospital may be the only realistically available treatment institution for a large number of its patients, and the reviewers' decisions that certain care is not reimbursable will reduce funds in a situation in which service cutbacks, if they occur, can only have an adverse effect on the quality and amount of care provided to the community. For the small urban or suburban hospital, PSRO-initiated funding reductions can lead to similar reductions in services, but the ultimate result may well be premature closure as a result of loss of community confidence and support. Because alternative treatment facilities are accessible, however, such closure would be likely to have a less severe impact on the surrounding community than the loss of an isolated (rural) hospital of similar size.

c. *Teaching Hospitals.* Medical-school-affiliated hospitals have traditionally supported teaching and research along with patient care. One consequence of this triple role is that in such hospitals most inpatient care is given by physicians-in-training (the house officers), who are accused of, or praised for, relying heavily on lab tests and complex diagnostic procedures both to establish the nature of the patients' diseases and to document thoroughness for their teachers, the attending staff. If PSROs do enough quality review, and that review is heavily process-oriented, the teaching hospitals' tendency to provide "aggressive" thorough work-ups may be financially rewarded. If PSROs' quality review is outcomes-oriented, teaching hospitals may also benefit, although possibly to a smaller degree. But if PSROs concentrate on cost-review, providing as few "medical necessity" loopholes as possible and interpreting length-of-stay and cost-of-ancillary-services guidelines rigidly, teaching hospitals (and, to the extent that it is funded by patients' medical fees, medical education as a whole) may be in trouble. On the average, teaching hospitals have longer lengths of stay and higher per-diem and ancillary-services costs than do non-teaching hospitals. If these longer stays and higher costs reflect a measurable extra severity and/or complexity of patients' illnesses, PSROs and medical-school-affiliated hospitals may be able to reach a mutually satisfactory accommodation to each other. If, on the other hand, the longer stays and higher costs reflect the provision of care which is useful for teaching but not necessary or useful for treatment, accommodation will be more difficult.

d. *Specialty Hospitals.* Maternity hospitals, clinical research centers, chronic-disease hospitals, inpatient psychiatric institutions, and, in fact, all specialty hospitals have one common concern about PSRO review: will the norms apply? The more a specialty institution's treatment patterns differ from those of the other hospitals whose statistics compose the PSRO's norms, the more likely it is that the institution will have to cope with denials or the threat of denials. But where deviance from the norm by a "normal" hospital can be presumed to signal at least a possibility of substandard care, such a presumption cannot be made in the reviewing of most specialty hospitals. In some cases, such as research centers, specialty hospitals will be treating patients for whose diseases neither norms nor standard diagnoses have been developed. The problems of PSRO review's effectiveness and applicability in such cases are obvious.

To a certain extent, all the foregoing concerns can be reduced to two: Will the hospital be financially crippled by the PSRO? And will the review system distinguish the hospital's patients' real needs if and when those needs are atypical? Review groups have to be aware of the immediate consequences of payment denials in varying societal contexts. If a small suburban hospital closes (however unlikely that may be), it may be only the hospital's employees who suffer, at least until they find new jobs. If a small rural hospital closes, it may be the entire community, and the effects may be permanent. If review labels a hospital as significantly deviant, and the hospital cannot change the review criteria or shift its accounting methods to recoup the lost money elsewhere, the consequences of continuing the review system will have to be assessed.

Fiscal Planning

A less obvious indirect effect than those outlined above, but one which has received some attention, is the improvement in fiscal planning that in theory can be better provided by a system of concurrent rather than retrospective payment denials. If a hospital administration knows that payment will not be forthcoming for patient x, it can encourage its medical staff to provide the least expensive acceptable treatment for that patient or even transfer him to another facility, thereby cutting losses. If, however, the hospital and its physicians always provide the least costly possible medical care, concurrent review is no better in this regard than is retrospective review, and the processing costs of concurrent review may be higher.

Capital Financing

Another problem for hospitals is the effect of PSRO review or other outside review on the hospital's ability to borrow money to finance capital improvements, new construction, and other long-term projects.

Private hospitals get long-term capital primarily from the following four sources: gifts (traditionally a major source but lately less available); the federal government (formerly via Hill-Burton); bank loans; and in some jurisdictions, tax-exempt bonds. One can hypothesize that gifts will continue to be given regardless of what the PSRO says about the hospital, provided that what it says isn't too damning. Hill-Burton loans were not statutorily tied to PSRO or UR approval; but with the advent of Health Systems Agency (HSA) planning, it is possible that the availability of government capital, if any, will depend in part on the institution's meeting minimal PSRO-monitored HSA standards.

Bank loans and tax-exempt bonds are both dependent on the good will of the financial community. The two most typical methods of bond financing are as follows. (1) The hospital "designs" the bonds and advertises their availability. Banking syndicates bid to "buy" the bonds, and the group that says it will assign the lowest interest rate wins the bidding. The bonds are then sold to the public by the winning bidder. The hospital pays off the bank, which then pays the holders. (2) The hospital designs the bonds, after which a banking syndicate negotiates with all the investors it can locate to get the best possible terms. Once the terms have been agreed upon, the syndicate buys the bonds and resells to the investing public as above.[17] Basically, what this means is that bankers and bond underwriters want to be assured that the hospital will be financially sound until the loan is paid off or the bonds retrieved. If those who are underwriting the loan or bonds think that PSRO review will have a negative financial impact on the hospital, either immediately or in the long run, they can refuse to take the risk, or they can demand more stringent conditions from the hospital in other areas of its operations in an attempt to reduce the likelihood of eventual insolvency. The impact of such conditions on patient care may not be knowable at the time the loan or bond agreement is signed.

It is possible, of course, that a hospital whose PSRO profile is very good may find itself in a comparatively advantageous position in the bond market or at the bank. Until the financial community develops confidence in PSROs, however, it is more likely that they will regard PSRO activities as a threat. If PSROs continue to concentrate on Medicare and Medicaid review and do not branch out into review of privately insured care, this will put hospitals which take high percentages of elderly and welfare-dependent patients at a relative disadvantage in obtaining long-term capital.

The Effect on Practitioners

The cost impact of peer review will ordinarily be less significant for physicians and other noninstitutional providers than for institutions. One of the reasons is obvious: physicians[18] will bear few of the direct costs of review themselves. Of all the direct costs, the only component likely to fall on the individual physician or other reviewed practitioner is the initial paperwork required by the data-processing system (e.g., notations in the chart to document justification for extended stay). There is, of course, an exception to this rule: in those areas where peer review groups ask physicians to donate their time to being reviewers and/or physician-advisors, some "salary" component will come from the physician volunteers.

The indirect cost impact on individual physicians is harder to assess. Within the PSRO program, review will initially focus on institutional care, so that only those physicians who own proprietary institutions, or whose salaries or fees come primarily from institutional services, will be at risk. It must be stated immediately that the risk is extremely small. In most areas of the country, PSRO review will be limited to Medicare and Medicaid patients, and will therefore have a limited impact at best. Most hospitals should be able to minimize even that impact by more aggressive patient management, changes in accounting procedures, and curtailment of unprofitable services.

Hospital-based physicians will be further insulated by the very nature of their relationship to their hospitals: because hospitals cannot exist without physicians' support (expressed as the willingness to admit and treat patients therein), the hospitals cannot afford to alienate those physicians by penalizing them financially when PSROs declare a treatment decision to be unacceptable, causing the hospital to be denied reimbursement for care which it is in the process of providing pursuant to the physician's orders. While it can be argued that the PSRO program's payment denials will be largely ineffective in changing unacceptable physician behavior until the physicians themselves feel the direct effect of those denials, the fact remains that as long as the hospital stands between the physician and the PSRO, there is little that the PSRO can do to insure that its message reaches those who actually make most medical treatment decisions.

Physicians who split their time between hospital and office will risk only their hospital-related fees, unless, after review, HEW removes them from program participation; physicians whose practices are entirely office-based may not come under initial PSRO scrutiny at all. Once PSROs begin to look at ambulatory care, any physician who sees patients covered by the program will be subject to denial of payment for any care he renders to those patients. This is, of course, the case at present for physicians who may be subject to peer review as part of a nonfederal reimbursement program—such as Blue Shield—wherever such a program provides for ambulatory-care review.

It should be noted that the threat of financial loss to private practitioners is rarely mentioned in the literature or testimony about the PSRO program, although PSROs' impact on hospital finances has been debated at some length. Reasons for this relative lack of concern may include the following:

- The medical community may realize that office-based care will not be widely reviewed for many years yet, even if a reasonable review methodology can be developed and agreement reached on the substantive norms or standards against which the ambulatory care would be judged. Ambulatory review, in other words, may not be seen as a practical threat.
- PSRO review is likely to remain limited, at least in the immediate future, to Medicare and Medicaid services, which are financially less significant for ambulatory care than for hospital services.
- Practitioners who fear or distrust the PSRO program's ultimate effects on the nation's medical system may feel that it would weaken their other objections if they focused on their own possible short-term financial losses.
- So far, PSRO review has had a limited financial impact on practitioners, and this experience may have mitigated the profession's initial fears.
- Physicians may feel that as long as the law requires that their work be reviewed by their fellows,[19] there is little danger that the review will be unnecessarily harsh. While few would be likely to agree, at least in public, with attorney Robert E. McGarrah, Jr., that "peer review is synonymous with self-protection,"[20] many no doubt feel that peer review, if not protective, at least is less likely to cause them financial harm than would any alternative cost control program.

Whatever the reasons, concern about PSRO review's impact on the profitability of private medical practice appears to be quite low. In the absence of adequate data on which to base an estimate of that impact, this is, perhaps, appropriate.

The Effect on Quality: The "Cost/Quality Tradeoff"

[Senator Wallace F. Bennett, Utah]: Do you know of any way in which your Department has indicated to [prospective] PSRO's [that] they should concentrate on cost savings at the expense of quality?
[Caspar W. Weinberger, Secretary of HEW]: No, sir.[21]

[Senator Herman E. Talmadge, Georgia]: Now you are operating . . . as something . . . that for all practical purposes is a PSRO . . . and it saved the Government and the State money?
[Kenneth A. Platt, M.D., Colorado Foundation for Medical Care]: Yes, sir.
[Senator Talmadge]: How about the quality of the service? Has it enhanced it or diminished it?
[Dr. Platt]: In our opinion, it has enhanced it. . . . First of all, any time a patient is placed in an institution which he basically should not be, that is in essence not quality practice. . . .[22]

As the above two excerpts from the Senate Finance Committee's Health Subcommittee 1974 PSRO oversight hearings illustrate, there are two aspects of the cost/quality debate, and both are of concern to those interested in the PSRO program. The first might be called the "practical" question: in a program where resources are limited, will the government's desire to control Medicare and Medicaid costs lead it to underfund quality review, leading to an actual reduction in quality, because higher-cost services cannot be "justified" within the review program? The second, or "theoretical," question is: can costs be limited or reduced without creating an inevitable adverse effect on the quality of the affected services?

The first question probably cannot be answered at this time. Certainly HEW's representatives, in both testimony [23] and written publications,[24] have indicated their desire not to shortchange PSROs' quality-monitoring functions. But it is also a fact that Congress has consistently appropriated less money for the PSRO program than HEW has requested in every year other than the first. In addition, while program appropriations may remain at relatively high levels as long as PSROs can document correspondingly higher cost savings in the Medicare and Medicaid programs, there will come a time when review has squeezed most of the "fat" out of the system, and it will become harder for PSROs to prove that their review is "cost-effective." One already hears allegations that length-of-stay reductions in PSRO-monitored hospitals "would have happened anyway" and are attributable to changing medical beliefs (i.e., that short stays are better for the patients) rather than to review-based reimbursement denials. Unless those who favor peer review can develop persuasive economic proof that PSROs save more than they cost, a period of severely reduced federal appropriations may be inevitable. If that happens, HEW may well direct PSROs to concentrate on cost monitoring in an effort to save the program from total dissolution.

The second question, whether cost control is compatible with high quality, can be answered with a limited but definite "yes." As Dr. Platt's answer to Senator Talmadge indicates, the experience of many Foundations for Medical Care and EMCROs has proved beyond reasonable question that whether one starts out trying to control costs or trying to improve quality, review will uncover instances where suboptimal practice and unnecessary expense coincide, and where control of one will lead to improvement in the other. As long as PSROs concentrate their quality-monitoring activities on those areas where quality improvement will reduce medical costs (e.g.: reduction of unnecessary hospitalization, reduction of premature hospital discharge where such discharges will lead to an increased readmission rate, improvement in antibiotic-prescribing practices), quality control and cost control will be partners rather than adversaries. In fact, it is possible to argue that for any given set of resource inputs (hospitals, insurance payments, federal subsidies, hours of physicians' time, etc.), there is some optimal level at which the amount of service can be maximized and the cost per unit of service minimized, and that PSRO review, intelligently performed, can point the country's medical system in the right direction and then help see that it stays there.

Even if one accepts the argument that PSRO-type review is capable of reconciling cost control and quality improvement, however, one must also understand that such reconciliation is not inevitable. PSRO can, by choosing the "wrong" quality-monitoring methodology, lead hospitals and physicians to adopt more elaborate and more expensive methods of diagnosis and treatment (processes of care) which are not justified by improvements in outcome (such as improved health or fewer readmissions). Similarly, adoption of a cost-monitoring system that does not permit reimbursement of care for atypical medical and sociomedical needs may well produce increased illness and concomitant increases in medical costs.

This latter possibility is apparently physicians' and hospital spokesmen's chief worry, but it must be pointed out, in fairness to the PSRO program, that PSRO review may be less likely than any other cost-control program to provide that undesired result. PSROs have a legal mandate to look at quality, whereas UR committees did not. It must also be remembered that federal and state governments could have simply cut Medicare and Medicaid reimbursement levels across the board rather than instituting a program that gives the medical profession a chance to make cuts where they will do the least harm. (If PSROs prove ineffective at controlling costs, as many have predicted, the federal government will quite probably change the law in just that way. During the recent recession, many state governments made as many cuts in their Medicaid covered service packages as the law allowed.) Are the medical professionals' worries about the cost/quality tradeoff justified? We do not yet know. But there is no justification for the position that PSROs *cannot* reconcile the difficulties. In theory and according to the preliminary evidence, it can be done.

CHANGES IN THE QUALITY OF CARE

Providers and consumers alike have expressed concern over PSROs' effects on the quality of medical care. Overall, the consumers' point of view appears to be that, cost effects aside, PSROs can potentially be beneficial in two ways: first, by monitoring care and educating or punishing substandard practitioners; and, second, by collecting data and making information based on that data accessible to consumers so that they can make more informed choices between physicians and hospitals. The theory is that such choices would result in greater use of and financial rewards to the better practitioners.

The consumer position supposes that PSROs will be able to make quality-related decisions based on accurate, quality-related information. To the extent that such information is not forthcoming and such decisions are not made, consumers are likely to suspect medical professionals of sabotage and noncooperation. To some extent, these fears may be justified.

One Massachusetts physician wrote in *PSRO Update:*

> Hospital clinical progress notes are already beginning to demonstrate a deterioration motivated by the physician's instincts for defensive coloration. . . . As PSRO establishes itself, we are going to see more and more of this deterioration . . . as physicians react in very human ways to surveillance. . . .[25]

The article goes on to compare reviewed physicians to public school teachers, whose written records are often devoid of any evidence of personal judgment, meaningful evaluation of their students, or utility to the reader or reviewer. While the analogy may be slightly extreme, one must admit that fear of adverse review decisions, occasionally coupled with the desire to hide major errors in diagnosis or treatment, could result in medical record distortions severe enough to invalidate any review program. In one notorious case,[26] a malpracticing physician not only falsified his progress notes, he discharged his patients from the hospital—whether they were ready or not, and all too often they were not—prior to their first mandatory length-of-stay review by a physician from the local Foundation for Medical Care. Many died as a result.

At present, however, such falsification appears to be very much the exception, and the effect of peer review on the quality of the medical record remains problematical. Debate about whether or not physicians are falsifying or gutting their records can only obscure the consumers' hidden assumption about peer review, one apparently shared by Congress at the PSRO program's inception: that adequate review methodologies and useful quality-related information are readily available.

Health professionals are less sure. PSROs, like computers, are only as good as the data fed into the system, and in the case of the PSROs, the quality-related data may be particularly unreliable.[27] If these fears are true—and evidence indicates that they are at least reasonable—the consequences of a PSRO's taking disciplinary action without extremely careful scrutiny at the peer review committee level and at any subsequent review, not to mention the consequences of release of identifiable information, including physicians' and hospitals' profiles, to the public, could be serious indeed. This is not to recommend that PSROs should sit back, accepting government money, and wait for someone to develop the perfect data abstract and/or the ideal review methodology. Rather, it is to suggest that the medical profession's concern that PSROs may adversely affect quality is not entirely groundless, and that PSROs should search for ways of performing review which will meet professionals' objections without emasculating the review process itself.

What are these professional concerns? When the subject of PSROs' nonfinancial effect on medical quality is raised, one is likely to hear about

- cookbook medicine
- weakening of other review efforts
- the stifling of medical-scientific progress.

For purposes of discussion, these and other complaints can be divided into two groups: those that deal with routine care, and those that deal with medical innovation.

Effects on Routine Care

Cookbook Medicine

In a statement that deserves praise for its lucidity and freedom from bias, Dr. Russell B. Roth, then president of the American Medical Association, explained to the Senate Subcommittee on Health during its 1974 PSRO oversight hearings why he thought there was a real danger of PSROs engendering overly routinized practice:

> ... Cookbook medicine would occur if there are indeed for each diagnosis a set of norms, and the understanding grows among all physicians that as long as their practice conforms ... fees will be paid and there will be no problem about peer review ... It seems to me that there will be a compulsion toward doing everything that the norm authorizes; the physician will feel if he does so he is secure, he is playing according to the Federal rules, and he will be paid, there will be no problems ... and it may even improve his legal status. ... .[28]

Dr. Roth was, of course referring to process standards, which at that time were the only type of quality-related criteria whose development was being considered or funded by HEW. (The AMA's official recommendation was that the PSRO statute be rewritten to make it clear that quality norms were to be used only as review "guidelines.") While Dr. Roth's stated concern was that cookbook medicine based on process standards would be more expensive than the medical system could handle, his comment and the comments of other witnesses and writers also carry overtones of two other concerns: loss of professional independence, and reduction of the physician's ability to tailor treatment to fit the special needs—medical, financial, familial, psychological, social, or whatever—of each patient.

Are these serious problems? To the extent that professional independence and the ability to deviate from the rules when necessary work for the patients' benefit, the answer is yes. However, professional independence can occasionally mask professional irresponsibility, and the ability to ignore accepted teaching can sometimes lead the overconfident practitioner to forget a necessary test or overlook a differential diagnosis that later proves correct. There are some—including, one presumes, most advocates of process criteria—who would argue that what American medicine needs is more "cookbook medicine," not less. The argument has been made that while it has not been proved that following process standards will lead to better treatment results (outcomes), there is likewise no proof that process standards are unrelated to outcomes. The main argument against process standards is that they will be expensive, not that they will ordinarily hurt the individual patient, except, perhaps, financially. The worst that can be said about process standards from a quality-of-care viewpoint is that in most cases the link between process and outcome has not been statistically validated. Would cookbook medicine be bad medicine? A nonprofessional observer might have to say that the answer is not yet in.

One's concern about process standards cookbooks would admittedly be greater if PSROs did not contain a peer review component, and if payment decisions were made by coordinators or computers on the basis of a process checklist which did not allow for the exercise of professional judgment and compassion. Such a system could, in fact, be implemented within Medicare and Medicaid, but PSRO, with its review committees and appeals processes, is not such a system. If the PSRO law is misinterpreted, or misused for the reasons Dr. Roth suggested, it is an unfortunate but avoidable consequence.

Weakening of Other Review Programs.

As we indicated in Chapter 1, PSRO review developed from earlier review programs, most of which continue to function at the present time. State medical and hospital licensure, JCAH accreditation, and various types of in-hospital quality review preceded PSRO and show every sign of maintaining themselves. Nevertheless, some commentators have expressed concern that PSRO review will supplant JCAH review, or weaken hospitals' commitment to other in-house quality-control operations, such as tissue committees, pharmacy boards, and transfusion review. Are these concerns well-founded? If they are, how serious would the consequences be?

To take the last question first: if PSRO review performs the same functions as other review efforts, and can do them more comprehensively or cheaply, there is no reason why the old systems should be preserved. To some extent, for instance, the JCAH's demand for in-hospital medical audit overlaps the PSRO law's quality-monitoring mandate, and one can assume that most hospitals and hospital-based physicians would object to doing twice as many audits as either program requires by itself. The solution to the conflict is obvious and has in fact been adopted by the PSRO program and the JCAH: both parties have agreed on a review methodology which will satisfy either program, and audits which follow the agreed-upon guidelines may be submitted to both the JCAH and HEW (via the PSRO) as evidence of compliance with their requirements. In general, it should be possible to meet PSRO requirements where they overlap with any other review requirements in the same way: have a single group of people perform the mutually-required review and report their results to all interested groups.

Thus we arrive at the first question, whether PSRO review will supplant other programs. The alleged problem appears to be a red herring.[29] Review programs, like many other organized human activities, have a momentum of their own, and it is probably fair to say that when purposes overlap, programs can be combined or the worse one phased out. When programs have sufficiently different purposes, it is probably safe to assume that both will continue to exist without adversely affecting each other.[30]

Peer Review and Medical Innovation

There are two ways in which PSRO-type review could affect the rate of change in the country's medical system. The first is by slowing or stopping what one might call systemic innovation, and the other is by restricting scientific (biomedical) progress.

Systemic innovation

The so-called "health care system" is, and probably always has been, in a state of constant change. As medical care becomes more complex, professional roles, treatment settings, and patients' expectations change. Perhaps the most obvious corollary to the rapid technological advance of recent decades has been the move of what had been home and office treatment to the increasingly laboratory-dependent office and hospital. Doctors' and nurses' jobs and training have become more science-oriented and fragmented; and whole new classes of technicians and paraprofessionals have been created to help keep the system running at a reasonable cost. One of the unforseen results of this trend is that many aspects of the traditional physician's professional and economic license-based monopoly have been ceded to the nurse and the physician's assistant. In the absence of a strong societal or professional reaction, one might expect this trend to continue. But the PSRO program gives physicians an opportunity to slow the rate of change, if not stop it entirely. As one observer commented,

> It is necessary to question PSRO reactions to innovative health programs or services that physicians may perceive as threatening their vested interests. Specifically, will PSROs allow nurses in the expanded role to practice if physicians feel threatened by them?[31]

The question could be asked as well for any profession within the system.

At the present time, the PSRO statue does not constrain PSROs from designing monitoring criteria which would effectively prevent hospitals from using nurse-clinicians, physicians' assistants, or even certain types of therapists in expanded roles. At the moment the problem is hypothetical, but the possibility exists that PSRO review could be abused by the physicians who control the program to serve their own economic purposes at the expense of other professions (and of the country as a whole), at least until HEW took action to stop such abuse. HEW's problem with this aspect of the review program is likely to be complex, because the abuse is likely to be subtle. The physicians who insist on physician input into or control over contested areas of care may be sincerely convinced that only such highly trained, expensive professionals can adequately assure an appropriate quality level. Physicians, like other professional groups, tend to equate the public welfare with their own professional welfare. The best solution to the impasse, if one develops, would be for HEW to mandate the use of outcomes standards in place of or along with process standards if it appears that process standards are being used to interfere with beneficial systemic innovations.

Scientific Progress.

In general, third-party reimbursement is not given for nonstandard treatments. While it is possible to laud this policy as a deterrent to malpractice, its effect on legitimate medical experimentation may not be so beneficial, either for the patient who is beyond the help of more conventional therapies or for society as a whole. PSRO review will make a somewhat sticky situation worse by identifying experimental treatments concurrently (before the chart can be changed, or items, such as the special consent form, conveniently misplaced). It can be argued that Medicare and Medicaid should not pay for human experimentation, even when that experimentation is intended to be diagnostic or therapeutic for the patient-subject. But the fact remains that a significant percentage of the costs of clinical experimentation are presently borne by federal and private insurers, contrary to their stated policies. If the PSROs' peer reviewers are sensitive to the need for clinical experimentation, they may be able to see that payment for experimental nonstandard care is not denied. Some commentators,[32] however, have expressed the fear that peer review is more likely to slow scientific progress in medicine than to advance it. It is not yet possible to say who is right.

PROFESSIONAL AUTONOMY, CORPORATE LIABILITY, AND PROGRAM CONTROL

No discussion of health professionals' concerns about PSROs and peer review would be complete without some consideration of the issues of professional control and independence. If any two statements can be called the leitmotif of antiPSRO thought, they are: "PSROs will invade privacy" and "HEW will end up telling us all how to practice medicine; HEW will practice medicine." The legal realities of the invasion-of-privacy argument are discussed in Chapter 6. But a word about professional autonomy is in order here. The rest of this chapter will also discuss two related issues: the way in which physicians, hospitals, and PSROs or other outside peer review groups are likely to share the responsibility for reviewing care (which touches on the issues in Chapters 7 and 8); and who ultimately controls the PSRO program itself, whether HEW, as many physicians charge, or the reviewed professions, as HEW claims. The remaining professional and nonprofessional concerns, with their large legal components, will be discussed in the subsequent chapters.

Professional Autonomy

Nonphysicians

The American Dental Association believes that the amendments [to the PSRO statute] we are suggesting should be accepted. To do otherwise is to subject a large segment of the dental profession to a highly regimented and stringent regulatory mechanism without any meaningful representation in its development and operation.[33]

Nurses cannot ... implement their standards of practice until each component is accepted by PSRO physicians ... The

PSRO law, as presently written, may herald the demise
of ... professional nursing as we know it today.[34]

These two warnings, the first by a dentist to the Senate Subcommittee on Health, the second by a sociologist to the American Public Health Association, are parallel reflections of a single major problem: health care practitioners who may be affected by PSRO decisions but who are excluded by law from PSRO membership fear the full implementation of PSRO review. "I have assumed all along that no doctor would review the work of a dentist, but that the PSRO would contract. ... We would have faced a serious problem if we had broken the line and opened the PSRO to anyone other than physicians and osteopaths. What about the physical therapists? What about the chiropractors? ..."[35] Senator Wallace Bennett, the law's sponsor, tried to explain to Dr. Sidney R. Francis, the dentist quoted above. In his plea, Senator Bennett comes close to admitting that the law itself provides no protection for the nonphysician practitioner ("... I have assumed all along ...") and that the only reason for limiting predeadline PSRO membership is to make the program more palatable to the physicians, without whose cooperation the PSRO program would be doomed.

The representatives of the dental profession on the stand that day responded by saying, "When it comes to the actual clinical review ... I think you are quite right; there is no question that most of these PSROs are going to make a contract ... that is not a serious concern to us ... The concern ... is that the PSRO ... is the place where ... the tone ... is going to be set. And we understand the practical problems ... but we feel ... we are in a slightly different position than perhaps some of the other groups to which you referred."[36] Or, in other words, it's not the reality ("actual clinical review") that is the primary importance, it's the sense of professional prestige ("the PSRO ... is the place where ... the tone ... is going to be set"); and being nice to us won't open the floodgates to all those people the physicians dislike; we can be differentiated from those other groups because we control a large component of the health care dollar ourselves; we're independently reimbursed.

In all fairness to the dentists, it should be pointed out that they are in the worst position of all nonphysician professionals vis-a-vis PSRO review: Medicaid and Medicare do reimburse dental care directly, and the reviewed dentist may have no hospital to stand between him and the PSRO, absorbing the financial impact of an unjust review denial. But the fact that PSROs' financial impact on nurse-clinicians and nurse-practitioners may be indirect (i.e., the hospitals, finding that they cannot successfully bill Medicare and Medicaid for expanded nursing services, might be tempted to cut off such services and substitute billable services in their place) does not make it any less severe. "Unlike physicians who want out . . . most nurses want in,"[37] reports a sociologist Miller, and the statement probably applies to every nonphysician professional whose income, professional role, and job satisfaction are at the mercy of the PSRO. Unlike the physicians, who fear only government interference, nonphysicians fear the doctors and the government together.

Physicians

In an article in the June 6, 1974, *New England Journal of Medicine,* Dr. Claude Welch argued that PSRO review was an inevitable outgrowth of the public's demand that physicians be publicly accountable for their decision: "The traditional independence of the profession clearly cannot exist in today's society."[38] Other medical professionals do not view the government's increasing interest in medicine as being either inevitable or desirable. "Rape, even if presented as motherhood, becomes rape again," [39] the *Wall Street Journal* reports one anti-PSRO physician as complaining.

The question of "Who's in charge?" has generated some of the greatest heat in the debate over PSRO. Even HEW itself is not immune. For example, in response to a question from Senator Talmadge during the 1974 oversight hearings, Secretary of HEW Weinberger implied that HEW lacked the power to involve itself in the standards-setting process: "That is in the local PSRO's. The power to set the standards and norms and criteria is, and in my opinion has to be, in the hands of local physicians . . ." [40] This is not strictly true, as Senator Bennett pointed out: "There must be some kind of a mechanism when it becomes obvious that this local system is falling down . . . ." [41] But even Senator Bennett's formulation, that ultimate control over PSRO standards rests with the NPSRC, a physician group, is not entirely correct. The Secretary of HEW, under the authority granted him in §1156(a), has the option of declaring unsatisfactory a local PSRO's standards. It is true that he cannot himself write substitute standards, but HEW and the NPSRC together can impose "such norms . . . as are approved" by the NPSRC. In most areas of PSRO operations, including reporting and sanctions, ultimate control rests in the hands of HEW totally without required NPSRC input.

And yet primary review must be done by the physician-controlled local PSROs. Who is in charge? While PSRO may look to some members of the medical professions like an unholy alliance between physicians and federal bureaucrats—or, in the more moderate words of New Mexico FMC president Hugh Woodward, MD., a "joint [effort] by a partnership arrangement between the government and the medical profession" [42] to the physicians, and to all individuals and institutions subject to review, the amount of government input into, and control over, the practice of medicine in America is not yet known. At present, HEW appears to be keeping to the minimal-interference tack first articulated by Secretary Weinberger, but policies can change. Nevertheless, if the federal presence in American medicine does increase, it will probably not be because of PSRO but rather because of the enactment of National Health Insurance in one form or another. Washington will exert more control over medicine by the way it tailors the benefits package than by any form of review.

Hospital Responsibility

Since 1966 and the Darling [43] decision in Illinois, American hospitals have begun to exert a tenuous control over their physicians. The Illinois courts articulated the then-revolutionary legal position that the modern hospital is not just a collection of buildings, it is an institution capable of forming an independent relationship with the patients who come to it for care; and that when the institution by its structure or historical behavior leads patients to have certain reasonable expectations, it must take steps when necessary to see that those expectations, including the belief that competent medical care will be provided in the emergency room and on the wards, are fulfilled. Although Illinois itself has backed off slightly from its comprehensive stand,[44] now holding that the hospital is only responsible for its employed physicians or those it assigns, but not for those earlier retained by the patient, most states which have considered the question of the hospital's liability—and therefore responsibility—for the malpractice of its medical staff have decided in favor of corporate liability.[45] The hospitals' need to monitor the quality of the work their physicians perform has grown apace. The JCAH's much-resented requirements for medical audits can be regarded as a response to a growing common-law trend, an effort to get hospitals to do what the law indicates they should before a malpractice lawsuit ensues.

Where does PSRO review fit into the hospitals' common-law review responsibilities? As previously indicated, JCAH, PSRO, and common-law review can be one and the same operation, and the hospital that does review for one purpose ought to be able to satisfy all three requirements. However, the PSRO's decision to refuse delegation to a hospital (or the hospital's decision not to seek it) could have one adverse legal consequence: if the PSRO itself, in performing nondelegated review, uncovers evidence of malpractice, and the involved physician and hospital are later sued, the hospital's legal claim that it was exercising "due care" in the choice and control of its staff could be considerably weakened by proof that the PSRO uncovered evidence which should have—and probably would have, had the hospital taken similar efforts to find out what was going on inside it—led to the hospital's investigating, and possibly disciplining, the errant physician. The nondelegated hospital has only two realistic legal alternatives: duplicate the PSRO's review, or ask the PSRO for all reports generated in the course of internal review, including physicians' profiles. Present HEW policy indicates that such reports can be released to the hospitals,[46] obviating the need for duplicative review; but until the regulations on data confidentiality are issued, the question remains legally open.

As with any legal responsibility, the assumption of a new duty carries with it an increased risk. If hospitals do receive PSRO reports, they will also have a duty to act on the given information. To have actual knowledge that one of your physicians is likely to commit repeated malpractice and to do nothing about it is marginally worse, in the eyes of most juries, than to have merely failed to take adequate steps to find out what your medical staff is doing.

Does PSRO review pose a threat to hospitals' increasing autonomy and control over the medical profession? The answer is a resounding "no." The real threat is that hospitals will not use the information that PSROs can make available to them, and will thereby shortchange their patients and subject themselves to increased legal risk.

Control of PSRO and Other Review Programs

As we have previously indicated, different review programs are appropriately controlled by different participants: medical licensure and hospital accreditation by the professions, hospital-based quality review by the hospitals and their medical staffs jointly, private peer review by the state and county medical societies, and PSRO by—whom? The most correct answer is that control of the PSRO program, although vested by the law in HEW, is at this time probably a joint effort. As long as HEW remains committed to the concept of peer review within the Medicare and Medicaid programs and itself lacks sufficient numbers of medically trained reviewers, control of the program will remain a joint venture. HEW appears at present to believe in medical peer review. Professional fears that the review program, and through it control of the medical profession as a whole, will be wrested from it, are at the very least premature.

NOTES

1. Such as the AMA, AAPS (Assn. of Am. Phys. & Surg.), CMS (Am. Assn. of Councils of Med. Staffs of Private Hosps.); see, in general, *Hearings on Implementation of PSRO Legislation* [PL 92–603] Before the Subcommittee on Health of the Senate Committee on Finance, 93rd Cong., 2nd Sess., pt. 1 (1974) [hereinafter 1974 Hearings].

2. E.g., 1974 Hearings at 399, 153: at 399, the AAPS characterizes HEW's position as being that PSROs will be run entirely by physicians (the characterization is right but HEW isn't) and then implies that the National Professional Standards Review Council will control the program (also not true); at 153 consumer representative Robert McGarrah says that HEW will be able to hide the names of disciplined physicians, whereas the Freedom of Information Act makes it very unlikely. A good example of emotionalism is the AMA's "Exorcising the Devil" speech in their anti-PSRO kit, referred to in the 1974 Hearings at 66.

3. Social Security Act §1156 (a), (b), and (c), 42 USC 1320c-5(a), (b), and (c).

4. 1156 (c) (1), 42 USC 1320c-5(c) (1).

5. Even salaried hospital-based practitioners may find that they cannot afford to help newly established PSROs unless their hospital can be reimbursed for their time or their salaries can be augmented. If the hospital absorbs the cost in any way, that amount must be added into the total national expenditure figures.

6. Larry Frederick, "PSROs: What Drs. Nationally Think of Them," *Medical World News* (October 25, 1974): 70.

7. According to a recent article in *Modern Medicine* (J. Snyder and R. Engelman, "PSROs—Time to Review the Peer Reviewers," Feb. 1, 1977, pp. 52-57), the controversial $35 limit will be raised "soon."

8. The requirement is implied in the statute and expressly stated in the accompanying report (S. Rept. No. 92-1230, 92nd Cong., 2nd Sess. (1972) [hereinafter Fin. Comm. Rept.]) at 261. See stat. §§1152 (c) (2) (42 USC 1320c-1 (c) (2)), 1152 (d) (42 USC 1320c-1(d)), and 1163 (e) (3) (42 USC 1320c-12 (e)(3)).

9. Fin. Comm. Rept. at 265.

10. *PSRO Management Information Systems Manual.*

11. Assuming, of course, that all PSROs start out from approximately the same position, which may not be a safe assumption. For their "baseline data" (against which they will ultimately measure their success or failure), PSROs will be dependent on other data-gatherers, such as state Medicaid agencies, regional planning groups (including federally funded Regional Medical Programs), private hospital associations, state rate-setting agencies, etc. If these other groups do not have the necessary data available or obtainable, the PSRO will have to collect and process the material for itself, possibly at a significant cost increase. On the other hand, if the PSRO does collect its own data "from scratch," it may be able to impose quality controls on that data which will render it more reliable, and possibly less expensive, in the long run.

12. The "criteria-development" process for UR consists primarily of the correlation of socioeconomic and medical data to lengths of stay, and the derivation of reasonable groupings. One need not know much about disease or cure to decide upon the points at which

one set of parameters rather than another should apply. For example, the decision to assign lengths of stay may be made on the basis of the number of co-morbid conditions as well as age (so that a 49-year-old man with two diseases in addition to his admitting diagnosis would receive a different LOS checkpoint than would a 49-year-old man with no other diseases and the same admitting complaint, and both would differ from a 69-year-old man similarly ill). This can be regarded as an economic policy decision (i.e., when is the number of categories sufficiently large to adequately discriminate between real groups of patients without being so large as to blur meaningful review distinctions because each group is too small to be statistically significant?) rather than a medical decision.

13. 1974 Hearings, at 193.

14. Id. See also the testimony of the CMS representatives at 298.

15. For example, see R. Egdahl, P. Gertman, et al., *Quality Assurance in Hospitals; Policy Alternatives* (New York: Springer-Vertag, Inc., 1976), p.10: "Effective PSRO activities may result . . . in . . . cost increases in some instances, because of improvements in quality. It is questionable whether the net effect will be a decrease in costs."

16. 1974 Hearings, p. 142. See also, Appel, Brook, "Quality Assessment: Choosing a Method for Peer Review," *New England Journal of Medicine* 288, no. 25 (June 1973): 1323.

17. See, in general, W. Gauntt, "Marketing Tax-Exempt Hospital Bonds: The Mechanics and Problems," *Tax-Exempt Financing of Hospitals and Health Care Facilities* New York: Practising Law Institute, (1975); pp. 148, 149.

18. The word "physician" will be used in some cases to include all similarly affected (noninstitutional) practitioners. The usage should be clear from the context.

19. §1115(c), 42 USC 1320c-4(c).

20. 1974 Hearings, at 152.

21. Id. at 20.

22. Id at 406.

23. Id. at 7-34.

24. W. Jessee, W. Munier, et al., "PSRO: An Educational Force for Improving Quality of Care, "*New England Journal of Medicine* 292 (1975): 668.

25. G. LeMaitre, "PSROs and the Violation of Privacy," *PSRO Update* 5 (September 1974): 3.

26. Gonzales v. Nork, Cal. Super. Ct. #228-566, Sacramento Co. (1973).

27. 1974 Hearings, p. 413, in material submitted by Dr. Kenneth Platt, of the Colorado FMC: "Our studies and experience . . . indicate that the data we need to accomplish medical care evaluation studies and the profiling required by PSRO . . . are not readily available in . . . current data systems."

28. Id. at 71.

29. Q: What's red, hangs on the wall, and whistles?
A: I don't know.
1st speaker: A herring.
2nd speaker: A herring? Are you crazy?
1st speaker: No, really: it's red because I painted it, and it hangs on the wall because I nailed it up.
2nd speaker: And the whistle?
1st speaker: Ah, I just put that in to make it harder.

30. E.g., medical licensure and PSRO or other peer review; in states where periodic re-licensure is the law, the licensure board could use PSRO review profiles rather than periodic reexamination if it chooses and if federal law permits, but it need not, and PSROs could do their review oblivious to the desires of the licensure board, or not. (p. 143).

31. M. Miller, "PSROs—Boon or Bust for Nursing," *Hospitals, JAHA* 49 (October 1, 1975): 82.

32. See, e.g., *PSRO Update* (June 3, 1975) at 6, quoting Dr. Selma Mushkin, or 1974 Hearings at 484, quoting Dr. William Blaisdell.

33. 1974 Hearings at 145.

34. Miller, at 84.

35. 1974 Hearings at 146.

36. Id. at 147.

37. Miller, at 81.

38. C. Welch, "PSROs—Pros and Cons," *New England Journal of Medicine* 290 (1974): 1319.

39. Spivak, *Wall Street Journal* (June 24, 1974), Col. 1, p. 1.

40. 1974 Hearings at 17.

41. Id. at 18.

42. Id. at 475.

43. Darling v. Charlestown Community Memorial Hosp., 33 Ill. 2d 326, 211 NE. 2d 253 (1965); lower court decision is reported at 50 Ill. App. 2d 253, 200 NE. 2d 149 (1964).

44. Lundahl v. Rockford Mem. Hosp., 93 Ill. App. 2d 461, 235 NE. 2d 671 (1968).

45. See, e.g., Darling, supra; Beeck v. Tucson Gen. Hosp., 18 Ariz App. 165, 500 P. 2d 1153 (1972); Pederson v. Dumouchel, 431 P. 2d 973 (Wash., 1967); Purcell v. Zimbelman, 18 Ariz App. 75, 500 P. 2d 335 (1972). But see, contra, Hull v. North Valley Hosp., 498 P. 2d 136 (Mont., 1972); Lundahl, supra.

46. Proposed regulations permitting PSROs to release "profiles, medical care evaluation studies and other pertinent information" to delegated hospitals can be found at 42 FR 1635 (January 25, 1977). If approved, the rule would become 42 CFR 101. 809(h). Proposed rule 42 CFR 101.710(e), mandating release of MCE results to involved hospitals, can be found at 42 FR 1630.

47. The interim final regulations issued on December 3, 1976 (42 CFR 101.1701 and 101.1702) deal only with nonidentifiable disclosures.

Chapter 4

The Constitutionality of PSROs

Is the government constitutionally able to mandate peer review? In two recent cases, two courts have indicated that the question is by no means settled. In the first case, the *Association of American Physicians and Surgeons et al. v. Weinberger,*[1] the United States District Court for the Northern District of Illinois (Eastern Division) found that the PSRO statute was constitutional in every respect. In the second case, *American Medical Association et al. v. Weinberger,*[2] Judge Julius Hoffman, in the same district, issued a preliminary injunction prohibiting the enforcement of certain parts of the utilization review regulations promulgated under Medicare and Medicaid. The injunction was upheld.

The enjoined sections would have required admission screening of all federally paid cases in acute-care hospitals. Such screening is permitted in the PSRO statute by Sections 1155(a) and 1156(d). While the AMA's lawsuit did not deal specifically with PSRO-mandated peer review, the type of utilization review it discussed is sufficiently close to PSRO-type review that the case can, and probably will, be taken as precedent, albeit nonbinding, if the question of the constitutionality of PSRO-mandated review is relitigated.

THE AAPS LAWSUIT

In its lawsuit, the American Association of Physicians and Surgeons (AAPS) alleged that the PSRO statute was unconstitutional on fourteen different grounds, embracing the first, fourth, fifth, and ninth amendments to the Constitution of the United States.

The AAPS's arguments can be divided into seven groups. The Association's major complaint was that the PSRO law unconstitutionally limited or deprived physicians of their right to practice their profession; their first, second, sixth, and seventh claims all bear on that question. Their other allegations were, basically, that the PSRO law

- unconstitutionally deprived patients of their right to treatment,
- unconstitutionally invaded physicians' and patients' privacy,
- was arbitrary, irrational, overbroad, and not justified by any compelling state interest,
- contained a section (§1160) which unconstitutionally denied due process to those to whom it applied,
- unconstitutionally granted judicial or quasi-judicial authority to biased groups or persons (the local PSROs), and
- contained a section (§1167) which was void in whole or part and which therefore exposed physicians to undue liability.

The best way to understand the case is to deal with each of these groups in turn. It should be noted that the government in its brief [3] also divided the AAPS's fourteen arguments into seven groups,[4] while the court used eight,[5] and that the groups do not correspond with those chosen here. Although it can be argued that any grouping of complaints tends to overlook the nuances of each individual argument, there is considerable overlap between and among various of the AAPS's arguments, and a separate discussion of each would tend to be unnecessarily repetitious.

The Right to Practice One's Profession

The AAPS's first, second, sixth, and seventh claims were that the PSRO law deprived them, entirely or partially, of the right to practice their profession, which is a property right, without due process of law: if true, this would be contrary to the fifth amendment. The District Court found that it was not: "This court finds that the challenged legislation is not so 'patently arbitrary and totally lacking in rational justification' as to be violative of the due process clause of the fifth amendment."[6] Two of the arguments raised by the AAPS in this context are interesting and deserve further discussion.

The AAPS's sixth allegation was that the PSRO law creates legal "presumptions" inconsistent with those allegedly raised by physicians' possession of medical licenses. Reduced to laymen's terms, this argument essentially means that once a physician is licensed to practice, he is invested with a property right which cannot be infringed or attacked in any way. Aside from the fact that the fifth amendment provides that property rights, or any rights, may be denied if due process is followed, this allegation is substantially similar to the first allegation made in the case. The court, while treating it separately, dealt with it summarily: "the Section . . . merely provides that practitioners must furnish evidence of their services in order to be compensated . . . accordingly, plaintiffs' contention . . . is without merit."[7]

The AAPS's seventh allegation was that enforcement of the PSRO law would "expose plaintiffs [physicians] to irreconcilable conflicts"[8] between their duty to be good physicians to their patients and their duty to the government, presumably to be law-abiding citizens. While it is possible to concede that the PSRO law does create some moral or emotional conflicts for physicians subject to it, any legal conflicts are far from "irreconcilable." In general, when there is an apparent conflict between two laws within a single jurisdiction, the more recent statute or case governs; the PSRO law is subject to the same sort of modification as other laws and itself modifies previous laws. Therefore, to take one example, even if a physician lives and works in a state in which the courts have held that physicians must maintain the confidentiality of patients' communications even against a subpoena, the PSRO law, if it postdates a court decision and if it preempts state law (and the federal courts can probably be relied on to find that it does preempt), will be held to override the earlier ruling. Therefore, there is no irreconcilable conflict.

It is particularly interesting that the AAPS treated this allegation as another fifth amendment due process problem. It is difficult to see how Congress' changing the law can be considered a denial of due process, even if some deprivation of property results from the change. Even more interesting is the court's refusal to deal with the allegation at length. Perhaps the judges felt it wasn't worth the trouble; or perhaps the AAPS's lawyers, seeing the essential weaknesses of the argument, refused to pursue it.

Deprivation of the Patients' Right to Treatment

The AAPS's third allegation was that the PSRO law interfered with the physician-patient relationship. The court held that the claim was "premature," especially in light of §1156's requirement that PSRO norms must allow for some regional variation.[9] While a first amendment argument, based on the 1973 abortion cases *Doe v. Bolton* and *Roe v. Wade*,[10] could possibly have been made, this allegation was argued strictly on fifth amendment grounds. On that basis, regarding the physician-patient relationship as essentially a property right of the physician, it is hard to see how the court could have decided otherwise, given its decision on the first argument in the case.

Invasion of Privacy

The first amendment was raised in the AAPS's fourth allegation: that the PSRO law infringed the patients' and physicians' right of privacy. Even here, however, the AAPS did not argue that the first amendment protected the physician-patient relationship itself from being scrutinized, but rather that confidential information derived from such scrutiny should not be divulged. The court rejected this argument, holding that "the challenged legislation in the instant suit seeks information for a legitimate governmental purpose."[11] Clearly holding to that branch of legal thought which says that privacy is a limited right, the court further found that "the manner in which the information is gathered and maintained is reasonable..."[12] and that "...the legislation contains provisions that properly balance the plaintiff's right of privacy with the government's interest in maintaining proper health care in an economical manner."[13] The court further held that the physicians bringing the lawsuit lacked standing to protect their patients' or potential patients' privacy rights.[14]

The AAPS also made a fourth amendment "privacy" argument: that the PSRO law's authorization of outside (governmental or quasi-governmental) inspection of physicians' records constituted "unreasonable search and seizure" of those records and was therefore prohibited. This is another argument which the court ignored. Basically, that oversight is probably justified; a number of cases exist which have held analogous record inspections to be "reasonable" and therefore permissible searches.[14] It is possible that if the plaintiffs had included some patients as well as physicians, or if the court had decided that physicians could assert their patients' claims, the judges would have given more consideration to a fourth amendment claim.

Overbreadth, Arbitrariness

The AAPS's fifth argument had three points: that the PSRO law was "an inefficient and unnecessary interference with their right to practice medicine,"[16] or, in short, was too broadly drawn for its stated purposes; that the law was arbitrary and irrational; and that there was no "compelling state interest" which would justify the law's enactment.

Responding to the AAPS's argument that the PSRO law was overbroad, the court found ample evidence in the legislative history that although the legislation is a "massive"[17] regulatory scheme, "the statute only provides standards for the dispensation of Federal funds...[and] does not bar physicians from practicing their profession."[18] Relying on a 1970 case which it believed "indicated that the overbreadth doctrine has little application to social welfare legislation,"[19] the court explicitly held:

> The [PSRO] law does not prohibit a physician from performing any surgical operations he deems necessary in the exercise of his professional skill and judgment. It merely provides that, if a practitioner wishes to be compensated for his services by the federal government, he is required to comply with certain guidelines and procedures enumerated in the statute.[20]

The court further held:

> It is true that there will exist economic incentive or inducement to participate in this program. However, such inducement is not tantamount to coercion or duress.[21]

These two findings are crucial to an understanding of the court's posture in this decision. They are primarily responsible for distinguishing the outcome of this case from that of the AMA's case, in which a different judge in the same court, dealing with similar legislation and identical precedent, reached an opposite result.

On the question of arbitrariness, the court disposed rapidly of the AAPS's arguments. It held that there was no evidence that the PSRO law created an "arbitrary and invidious discrimination"[22] as does a statute distinguishing between people on the basis of race, and that there was no evidence of denial of procedural due process in the PSRO legislation. In fact, the court found that §1159 of the PSRO law (42 USC 1320c-8) gave more than adequate due process guarantees under the fifth amendment.[23]

Against the AAPS's claim that there was no compelling state interest to justify the passage of the PSRO law, the court found that the statute's cost-control purpose saved it from unconstitutionality, as did the voluntary nature of physicians' and patients' participation in Medicare and Medicaid.[24] Admitting that the PSRO law "comes in close proximity to the rights of ... physicians ... in the Medicare and Medicaid programs, yet, there must be a balancing between those interests and the government's interests in providing and maintaining medical care to those most in need of it."[25] The court also properly warned that its decision touched only the constitutionality of the statute "on its face" and that it was not discussing any particular regulatory application of the statute. The court reminded the litigants that the mere unwieldiness of any bureaucracy which might be created was a problem for the legislative branch of government, not the judiciary.[26]

§1160 and Due Process

The AAPS's eighth allegation was that §1160, which itemizes physicians' duties, and therefore the PSRO law as a whole, was unconstitutionally vague. Here again, the court found that "plaintiff's argument appears premature,"[27] but it also said, in dicta, that "Congress did not stray beyond the permissible boundaries of the Constitution" in relying on such undefined terms as "medically necessary ... professionally recognized ... [and] proper care."[28]

The court did not deal specifically with the AAPS's ninth claim, that §1160(b)'s sanctioning procedures were also so vague as to constitute a denial of due process. However, in its discussion of the AAPS's claims of unconstitutional denial of the right to practice one's profession, the court did suggest that any infirmities in §1160's sanctioning procedures was cured by §1159's guarantees of legally adequate hearings and appeals.[29]

Delegation to Biased Groups

The AAPS's eleventh allegation was that the PSRO law was an unconstitutional delegation of authority to potentially biased private organizations. Relying on precedent, the court held that:

> It has been held permissible for agencies of the federal government to contract with private organizations in order to have such organizations perform governmental functions as long as the particular administrative scheme provides for a hearing of the determinations made by those private organizations.[30]

The court—and the government, in its brief—gave short shrift to the AAPS's allegation that delegation of judicial authority to private groups is unconstitutional if a possibility exists that the groups will be unavoidably biased in their judging. Both apparently felt that the AAPS had not provided a sufficient factual basis to support what in other circumstances might have been a correct legal theory.

§1167

The AAPS's twelfth, thirteenth, and fourteenth complaints were that Congress lacked the authority to change state law as it arguably did in

§1167 of the statute, or, alternatively, that if Congress had not changed the law, it subjected plaintiffs to unnecessary legal risk. The court found, first, that the plaintiff physicians were not the proper parties to challenge that provision, as they lacked standing; and, second, that the claim was again premature. The court's decision was correct on the issue of standing. Reduced to laymen's terms, what the court was saying was that if the grant of immunity from liability could be made to stick in a malpractice case, it would not be the physician who was harmed.

It is interesting to note that in justifying the PSRO law, the court looked upon it as the "first medical utilization review program that is national in scope."[31] The court shied away from looking at the quality monitoring aspects of the PSRO legislation. Considering that these were argued only in a fifth amendment property-rights context, it is perhaps understandable that the court was not impressed by the AAPS's argument that the PSRO statute presented a threat in this regard. Yet, as we will see, it was essentially the argument that review would deprive patients of the access to high quality care that was dispositive in the case of *AMA v. Weinberger.*

THE AMA's CASE

In trying to stop the UR regulations which had been published as final on November 29, 1974, the American Medical Association made two basic substantive arguments. The first was that the UR regulations interfered with physicians' and patients' constitutional rights to practice medicine and to receive medical treatment (first, fifth, and ninth amendments). The second argument was that the UR admission review regulations violated §1902(a)(9) of the Social Security Act,[32] and that HEW, in drafting the regulations, had exceeded the authority granted to it under the authorizing legislation,[33] and in any case had violated fifth amendment due process requirements and the Administrative Procedures Act.

Insofar as the second argument deals with the statutory basis of the UR regulations, it need not concern us here, because that basis differs from the statutory basis of PSROs and the arguments which can be made against one cannot be made against the other. The argument that HEW has violated due process requirements and the Administrative Procedure Act may be raised against any given set of PSRO regulations, but are not pertinent to the question of whether or not the statute itself is constitutional. Therefore, the AMA's lawsuit is relevant to the PSRO program only in its first arguments that the law mandating review is constitutionally infirm.

On the question of the constitutionality of the UR regulations, the AMA's case can be divided into patients' rights arguments and physicians' rights arguments.

The AMA alleged that the UR regulations unconstitutionally abridged patients' first and ninth amendment right to treatment as well as the fifth amendment "protection of 'life, liberty and property'."[33] The association argued that *Doe v. Bolton*[34] and *Griswold v. Connecticut*[35] had incontrovertibly established the right to treatment as absolute. The AMA did not reach the question of how "fundamental" the right was, but chose rather to argue that the federal government's "interest in conserving the expenditure of governmental funds ... is neither substantial nor compelling"[36] as a matter of law. The association also argued that the regulations were in fact incapable of generating the cost savings they were allegedly designed to produce:

> Thus, the Secretary's decision to interfere with all hospital admissions by subjecting them to wholesale review rather than focusing on precisely identified areas where medical resources are particularly scarce or where the danger of unnecessary admissions is particularly great not only eliminates any possibility that cost savings will be effected by the regulations but also constitutes an overly broad interference with constitutionally protected rights.[38]

In other words, the AMA was arguing that the PSRO program had no basis in law or in fact for abridging the rights to give and receive treatment.

In their attack, the AMA's lawyers distinguished preadmission certification from concurrent and retrospective review. While preadmission certification was repugnant to the first, fifth, and ninth amendments because of overbreadth and lack of relationship to the law's stated purposes, they argued, concurrent and retrospective review were unacceptable infringements of physicians' and patients' first amendment rights because such review would exert a "chilling" effect on the treatment process.[39] This process, they claimed, is at least partially protected by the constitutional guarantee of free speech. Against a possible defense theory that participation in Medicare and/or Medicaid constituted an automatic partial "waiver" of one's first amendment rights, the AMA argued that Congress and the courts were constitutionally prevented from being able to make receipt of government money conditional upon the surrendering of a constitutional protection.[40] In addition, the AMA argued that the "waiver" theory was invalid when applied to nonfederally-reimbursed patients to whom UR would be applied.

Judge Julius Hoffman, hearing the arguments during the AMA's plea for a temporary injunction against enforcement of the UR regulations (during which the plaintiffs must prove only that they could possibly win a full-scale lawsuit, and that if the court does stop the defendant first, the plaintiffs will be so badly harmed that winning will be useless to them), professed not to be entirely convinced by the AMA's interpretation of previous cases:

> The court notes . . . that the consequence of violating the state abortion statute in *Doe v. Bolton* . . . was criminal prosecution of the . . . doctor, not denial of reimbursement under a social welfare program.[41]

Judge Hoffman also noted that some of the facts upon which the AMA relied, even if true, were probably irrelevant.[42] The court's ruling was based on the following findings:

> . . . According to the testimony . . . the practical effect of the regulations is to deny admission, even if the terms of the regulations do not,[43] . . . There is no indication that an over-65 indigent recipient of Medicare or Medicaid, if not admitted under these programs, could otherwise pay for the hospitalization prescribed . . . [The] potential injury to the patient's health may be irreparable . . . [44]
>
> The wiser exercise of this court's discretion [when a preliminary injunction is being requested] is the issuance of [the injunction] pending disposition on the merits. The risk of irreparable injury to the health of patients outweighs any hardship to defendant [HEW]. . . .[45]

The circuit court to which HEW appealed upheld Judge Hoffman's order:

> The only question before this tribunal is whether the trial court committed an abuse of discretion in issuing a preliminary injunction. . . . Our review of the case, as presented thus far, leaves us with the impression that the plaintiffs [AMA] could ultimately succeed. Yet, a full trial on the merits . . . may lead to a different conclusion . . . we do not intend to express any view on the . . . merits of plaintiffs' claim. . . . AFFIRMED.[46]

The full trial that the district and circuit courts had anticipated was never held. HEW withdrew the regulations shortly after the circuit court announced its decision, and the withdrawal removed the "controversy" that the law demands must exist before litigation will be considered proper.

Application of the AMA's case to the question of the PSRO program's constitutionality is tricky, partly because of the lack of any decision on the merits of the AMA's case, and partly because there are some serious differences between the legal/constitutional status of the UR regulations and the PSRO statute. Perhaps the most serious difference is that, in the trial court's opinion, there was a real concern that the UR regulations contravened the spirit and letter of the statute under which they were ostensibly enacted:

> Quite clearly, one of the principal purposes of the regulations is to reduce rapidly rising costs of federal health insurance. Equally clearly, however, the larger purpose of . . . the enabling legislation is the delivery of medical services to those otherwise unable to obtain them. If twenty-four hour review of admissions [frustrates treatment] . . . this larger goal is thwarted.[47]

This argument is not available to those who would attack the PSRO program. PSROs have a clear statutory mandate to do exactly that which the AMA's district court stated was probably impermissible for the UR program. Any attack on the PSRO program will have to prove that cost cutting in Medicare/Medicaid is actually unconstitutional rather than merely illegal. While this sounds difficult, it is—at least for some aspects of the PSRO program—not necessarily impossible.

THE CASE FOR AND AGAINST PSRO

What arguments can be brought against the PSRO program? Despite the Seventh Circuit decision upholding the PSRO law, the question of the constitutionality of the statute should not necessarily be considered closed, and the regulations which HEW will issue will themselves be subject to attack on the grounds of unconstitutionality and certain other forms of illegality.

The basic arguments against the PSRO statute and/or regulations are: impermissible interference with protected rights, vagueness,[48] overbreadth, and impermissible delegation to private parties.[49]

Denial of Protected Rights

Does the PSRO law unconstitutionally interfere with anyone's constitutional rights?

The Constitution does permit infringement of constitutional rights in certain circumstances, such as whenever a more fundamental right is at stake. To determine whether or not specific rights have been unconstitutionally invaded is therefore a two-step process: one must first see if any constitutionally guaranteed rights are affected by the program, and one must then ask whether or not there is an impermissible infringement of any of those rights. It is probably fair to say that there are only three constitutional rights which the PSRO law can be seriously argued to infringe: the patient's right to treatment; the doctor's right to practice his profession; and the patient's, and perhaps remotely the physician's, right to privacy.

If the right to receive treatment, the right to practice one's profession, and the right to have some sort of privacy in the giving or receiving of treatment do exist under and are protected by the Constitution, the question would then become: can the federal government limit or deny those rights under the circumstances or by the methods involved in the PSRO law? The answer may well be "yes."

The Patient's Right to Treatment

The Supreme Court's 1973 abortion decisions, *Doe v. Bolton*[50] and *Roe v. Wade*,[51] may or may not have established a constitutionally based right to medical treatment. This right, if it exists, is based on the first, fourth, fifth, ninth, and/or fourteenth amendments.

Does the "right to treatment" exist? Certain language in the Roe and Doe decisions implies that it does, at least in one highly controversial instance:

[the] right of privacy ... is broad enough to encompass a woman's decision whether or not to terminate her pregnancy.[52] [Committee approval] substantially [limits] ... the woman's right to receive medical care in accordance with her ... physician's best judgment. ... [53]

The language seems clear. But there is no mention in the Constitution of either privacy, abortion, or medical treatment as a protected right, unlike the clear rights to freedom of speech, press, assembly, and religion, maintenance of a state militia, fair trial, due process of law, etc. Where does the Court's position come from?

The answer depends, to some degree, on which Justice's opinion you read. Justice Blackmun, speaking for the majority of the Supreme Court in Roe, said that the Constitution need not be explicit:

> In a line of decisions . . . the Court has recognized that . . . a guarantee of certain areas or zones of privacy does exist under the Constitution. In varying contexts, the Court or individual Justices have . . . found at least the roots of that right in the First Amendment, . . . in the Fourth and Fifth Amendments, . . . in the penumbras of the Bill of Rights, . . . in the Ninth Amendment, . . . or in the concept of liberty guaranteed by the first section of the Fourteenth Amendment . . . only personal rights that can be deemed "fundamental" or "implicit in the concept of ordered liberty" . . . are included in this guarantee of personal privacy.[54]

What is happening, of course, is that the Supreme Court is in the process of creating and defining a right, and has not yet settled upon a legal rationalization for it; nor has it yet defined those limitations beyond which the right will not extend.

It appears clear, at this time, that the Court, despite its frequent references to the "right of privacy," intends to create that right by finding instances in which the Constitution's provisions can be regarded as protecting some plaintiff's interest in maintaining privacy, and interpreting the provisions to fit. It is probably fair to say that even if the right to privacy, as a whole, does not yet have complete constitutional protection, the right to treatment has been given a reasonably firm constitutional footing by the 1973 abortion decisions. Whether that right is based on the first amendment (protecting freedom of communication between doctor and patient), fourth amendment (the right to be "secure" in regard to oneself and one's "papers and effects"), or fifth amendment (no deprivation of life or property without due process of law) is probably less important than determining how "fundamental" that right to treatment is. Although the Supreme Court explicitly did not decide the issue in the abortion context,[55] the question will be crucial to any litigation involving the validity of the PSRO law.

The first problem, for those who would attack PSROs' ability to deny payment for certain treatments on the basis of concurrent review, is that the Supreme Court's 1973 decisions did not merely leave the door open on the question of fundamentality, they provided at least two sets of opposing dicta. On one hand, the Court promised that only fundamental rights could be considered subject to constitutional protection of privacy, and then said that a woman's "right to receive medical care" was, at least in some respects, protected against a state's interference.[56] On the other hand, the decisions explicitly warn that the privacy-related right "to do with one's body what one wishes"[57] can be severely limited.[58]

If the right to treatment is fundamental, the state and federal governments will be required to have a "compelling state interest" before attempting to limit the free exercise of that right in any way. If the right is merely ordinary, the only requirement is that the limitation be based on bare rationality and any legitimate purpose. In Roe, the Court held that the state's interests must be "important"[59] if it is to abridge the right to do what one will with one's (and one's fetus's) life or health. This would indicate that the right of rational self-determination in the medical treatment context is less than fundamental and yet more than ordinary. Nevertheless, there are warnings, in Doe v. Bolton, that a "reasonable" statute could well pass constitutional scrutiny when the right to treatment is involved.

Consider the parallels between the Georgia antiabortion statute and the PSRO law. Both attempt to limit the patient's right to treatment by requiring that one or more physicians approve the treating physician's diagnosis that a need exists for a given prescribed treatment, and both require that treatment be given in an appropriate facility.[60] Although both requirements were held to be constitutionally impermissible in an abortion law, the reasons for the Court's holding were that the statutes were not justifiable on the basis of the limited evidence[61] (in the case of matching facility to treatment) produced by the state, were overbroad[62] and were not rationally connected to the patient's needs[63] (in the case of the two-physician concurrence).

In other words, if the government can prove in any court defense of the PSRO program that satisfactory evidence exists that certain medical procedures can, and for financial reasons ordinarily should, be limited to certain facilities, it will be able to maintain that aspect of the law. If the government can prove either that available professional disciplinary activities have not been adequate to reduce the "abuses" at which the PSRO law is aimed, or that its own sanctions are appropriately drafted and are rationally connected to the allowable purpose of saving government money, it should be able to maintain that aspect of the law as well.

Because the Doe and Roe cases can be read as establishing two, or even three, positions on the fundamentality of the right to treatment, those who dislike the PSRO law would do well to find an alternative legal method of limiting the impact of PSRO operations. Is such an alternative available? Maybe. If anti-PSRO litigants can prove that the PSRO law is, in intent or effects, "aimed" at a "suspect category" of patients, the government will again be held to a "compelling need" standard. Race,[64] sex,[65] and economic class[66] have all, at one time or another, been considered suspect categories.

While it would be extremely difficult, if not absolutely impossible, to argue that the PSRO statute was intended to limit the availability of medical care for the black and poor, it may be somewhat easier to prove that the statute's effects are unacceptable. The recipients of Medicare and Medicaid are, on the whole, among the nation's most disadvantaged economic groups. While it is unlikely that a court would be willing to find on that basis alone that the PSRO law was unconstitutional, proof that in fact the program operated to deprive these people of their rights, and that no such restraints had been placed by the government on richer (or younger, or whatever) persons' exercise of their rights to treatment,[67] might well convince a court that the government had to produce a compelling justification for the PSRO statute and regulations. Against this line of argument, the government's defense might be that PSRO is a component of a "social welfare" program, and therefore that its justification need merely be ordinary. The merits of this argument will be discussed in the section on "overbreadth."

One other aspect of the right-to-treatment question must be mentioned. Whether or not the right to treatment is fundamental, and whether or not the government's justification of the PSRO law and PSRO review must provide a compelling state interest, the right to treatment itself may be limited by the Roe court's presumption that wide latitude in medical judgment "operates for the benefit, not the disadvantage, of the [patient]."[68] Roe v. Wade can therefore be read, independently of all the considerations discussed above, as establishing a universal right to treatment (fundamental or not), or a right to treatment only when a reasonable person could safely presume that treatment will be beneficial, or no right to treatment at all. If the courts accept the first reading, PSRO review could be held to be as constitutionally unacceptable as the three-physician screening panel required by the Georgia abortion law. If the courts accept the second reading, PSROs would not be constitutionally prohibited from seeking to separate the physician whose quality of care was judged to be substandard from the patients whom he seeks to treat and who seek treatment from him. If the courts accept the third reading, all review is desirable.

The Physician's Right to Practice His Profession

The practice of a profession is a source of wealth. It is also a property and as such is protected by the fifth amendment's due process guarantee.

In every state where the question has been argued, it is settled law that the medical license is a property which gives its holder a "right" to rely on its continued use and possession.[69] In the federal court system, therefore, when right-to-practice cases are litigated, the question of whether such a right exists independent of state law under the U.S. Constitution has never had to be reached. The basic presumption is that the federal Constitution does not create any substantive rights beyond those established by state law, except where constitutional rights are expressly stated or can be found by the courts.

The right to practice one's profession is not absolute. All states which grant medical licenses also provide for their removal in those cases where the physician's practice does not meet state standards. Granted that possession of a medical license gives the owner a property right in his professional practice which cannot be taken away or interfered with without full due process proceedings, one should not mistakenly assume that this implies that the right to practice cannot thereafter be revoked or limited. The right to practice one's profession is, in part, a right to have due process during revocation or limitation proceedings. In general, allowing for state-to-state variations, other rights which inhere in the license include the following: the right to make diagnoses and to prescribe treatment, including drugs and other therapeutic medications or regimens; the right to deliver babies; the right to represent oneself as being a physician; and the right to receive payment or other remuneration for any or all of those activities. PSRO review, if it results in a decision not to pay a physician for doing any of those things, does interfere with professional practice. The questions must, therefore, be: can PSRO interference be justified? If the interference is justified, do PSRO review, hearings, and appeal processes meet fifth amendment due process standards?

PSROs' interference with professional practice can be constitutionally justified on a number of grounds. To the extent that professional practice is a property right, the government need only show that it is providing due process to the aggrieved practitioner. To the extent that the right to practice is derived from the patient's right to receive treatment, the government may have to show that it has sufficient justification, as well as providing due process and meeting other constitutional tests, some of which will be discussed later in this chapter. But once the government has met its burden of proof in regard to the privacy-related questions, interference with professional practice would have to be considered fully constitutional.

As for the second major question, the answer is probably a resounding "yes": PSRO procedures do meet fifth amendment due-process standards. While the question is one of fact as well as law, it is hard to fault the PSRO statute on any ground related to fairness or procedural adequacy (other than possible vagueness, which will be discussed). This does not mean, of course, that any or all of HEW's regulations of PSRO procedures will necessarily pass constitutional scrutiny; and it certainly does not mean that all PSROs will in fact proceed against those they review in a manner which satisfies the fifth amendment. What is difficult to imagine would be a court's finding that the PSRO statute, as presently in force, unconstitutionally interferes with professional practice.

Patients' and Physicians' Rights to Privacy

In the context of PSRO operations, the right to privacy, to the extent that it exists at all, may be breached in two separate ways. The first, and more obvious, is by the PSROs' ability, however limited, to publish data about their patients, hospitals, or physicians. The second is by the PSROs' ability to gather such data.

On the question of publication (i.e., by the review coordinator to the PSRO and/or by the PSRO to other parties), it is not clear that the patient's interest in the confidentiality of the information in his medical record is a protectable "right." The legal ramifications of the various publication options available to PSROs can be found in Chapters 2 and 6.

Pertinent to the question of data gathering is the 1973 abortion cases' clearly articulated position that review—or at least screening prior to treatment—may be an unconstitutional invasion of the patient's right to treatment, as discussed above. As the right to treatment is probably constitutionally indistinguishable from the right to privacy in any fact situation involving PSRO review or data-gathering activities, further discussion of the legal issues at this point is unnecessary. It should be noted again, however, that the physician's right to privacy rests on an even less firm constitutional footing than does the patient's; this is true whether one refers to the right to privacy in terms of publication of data or the right to privacy in terms of the right to give treatment.[68]

Overbreadth

Assuming for the sake of argument that the government has legitimate interests which it sought to protect by enacting the PSRO law, is that law the least drastic available means to protect those interests or regulate the conduct of those involved?

In passing laws the government is not permitted to infringe anyone's pre-existing legal or constitutional rights unless such infringement is necessary for the law's successful operation. If the law infringes unnecessarily, it is considered "overbroad."

In the medical context, *Griswold v. Connecticut*[71] furnishes a practical example of the application of the overbreadth doctrine. There, the U. S. Supreme Court, overturning a physician's conviction for violating a Connecticut anticontraceptive statute, held that while the state had a right to regulate the manufacture and sale of contraceptives, its prohibition of their *use* unnecessarily invaded spouses' right to marital privacy and their physicians' right to render aid to them when asked.

It is not clear how the overbreadth doctrine will or should be applied to the PSRO program. A long line of cases holds that the doctrine should not usually apply to "welfare" cases, and the PSRO statute can certainly be regarded as falling within the broad category of welfare law. It may seem odd, at least to nonlawyers, that "welfare rights" can be more easily abridged than other types of rights, but there is a legal rationale for distinguishing "welfare" cases from other types when applying the overbreadth rule.[72] That rationale rests on the distinction between "rights" and "privileges" under law.

The question, basically, is: Whose property is Medicare? The traditional legal theory is that Medicare (and Medicaid) payments are the property of the government, which can bestow them where it sees fit; i.e., the executive branch can do anything with the money that the relevant statutes and cases permit. There are limitations to the government's freedom other than those which it imposes on itself by statute. The Supreme Court has held, for example, that the due process clause[73] prohibits arbitrary withholding of Social Security benefits,[74] although it remains up to the courts to decide what constitutes arbitrariness in each litigated case. There are no simple yardsticks.

Some have argued that the traditional view is wrong, and that Medicare and all other "welfare" payments should be considered the property of those who can claim beneficiary status under the law. Perhaps the most persuasive exposition of this second view is Charles Reich's 1964 article, "The New Property,"[75] in which he argues that all forms of property are equally dependent on government action for their existence, and that to regard the Medicare beneficiary as receiving money as a "privilege" rather than a "right," is the same as saying that a landlord holds his real property subject to easily revocable government license rather than by right, or that the "right" to practice a profession is in fact a "privilege." The chief distinction between a right and a privilege is the ease with which the government can revoke each, including, for example, the amount and type of legal process which is "due" to the subject of the revocation proceeding.

Reich's argument is that in modern America, increasing numbers of people are becoming increasingly dependent on government largesse (such as welfare, licenses to operate broadcasting facilities, licenses to drill for offshore oil, et al), and that the courts should make it as hard as possible for the government to revoke what it has given out. While most courts have not fully embraced this argument, it has influenced a line of cases which can be read as holding that when the government's largesse is crucial to the beneficiary's survival, (e.g., having a place to live), full constitutional protection must be given that beneficiary before the largesse is revoked.

Ordinarily, health care would be regarded as the equivalent to health or life itself, the rights to which should be invaded narrowly or not at all. One can argue, however, that the PSRO statute is directed at health care that itself infringes the patient's health or jeopardizes his life. Those who seek to overturn the PSRO statute on overbreadth grounds would therefore be well advised to concentrate on the allegedly inevitable side effects of any review program, including the possibility of life-threatening incorrect no-pay decisions, rather than on the existence of review itself.

In the PSRO law, the specific provisions most likely to be attacked on overbreadth grounds are those permitting preadmission screening. To complicate matters for HEW, however, it is also possible to argue that the requirements for admission screening and periodic recertification are equally unnecessary to effect the stated statutory objective "to promote the effective, efficient, and economical delivery of health care services," at least for most providers. The reason for this can be found in the statute itself. If the PSRO confines itself, as the law appears to require, to making review decisions on the basis of accepted regional norms, the majority of its physicians will, by definition, never be adversely affected. Even if the PSRO makes its judgments on the basis of professionally developed standards, a practical assumption would be that those standards were acceptable to at least the majority of PSRO physicians, even if a somewhat smaller number of them actually met the standard. Universal screening would therefore appear to be utterly unnecessary except for the purpose of identifying deviant practitioners. Such physicians can be identified just as quickly by retrospective review as they can be by admission, preadmission, or concurrent review. Because preadmission screening will probably interfere with some patients' ability to get treatment of the type and at the time and place which they and their physicians have agreed upon, and because all three types of review will call for significant expenditure of federal funds and private parties' time and effort, an argument can therefore be made that only after retrospective review has identified those persons or institutions who seek to promote ineffective, inefficient, and uneconomical[77] health care should the more constitutionally repellant review procedures be instituted. Where there is factual proof that less invasive procedures have failed and will quite probably continue to fail, the government may possibly be entitled to use the more invasive procedures in pursuing its legitimate and compelling interests. The opposing argument can be made that use of a retrospective screening process will guarantee an initial period during which deviant practitioners can continue to be ineffective, inefficient, and uneconomical, but the law appears to demand that when constitutional rights are being invaded, the government must supply proof that such a delay would so hamper its compelling interest in saving money that the courts would be prohibited from permitting retrospective screening.

It is apparent that the drafters of the PSRO statute recognized that preadmission screening was probably not universally desirable, and, indeed, preadmission screening is the most constitutionally repellant review procedure. It is possible that the implication of §1155(a) that other methods must be tried first will protect preadmission screening from being found unconstitutional. It is also clear that invasions of privacy and interference with professional practice will take place no matter which screening procedure is used. If one grants that some form of screening is necessary to protect federal expenditures for health care, it is hard to invalidate admission screening or concurrent recertification on any overbreadth grounds other than the purely economic. No one has ever successfully argued that courts have a right to force Congress to make useful expenditures of taxpayers' money.

Vagueness

If a statute or regulation is so badly drafted or so general in its terminology that a reasonable reader would have trouble understanding what conduct it was that the drafters sought to prohibit, the statute or regulation will be struck down on the grounds that enforcement would deny the sixth amendment right "to be informed of the nature and cause of the accusation" being made against the defendant or the fifth amendment right to due process. Vagueness, like beauty, is often in the eyes of the beholder, and the situation is complicated by the legal doctrine that a statute or regulation need not contain all of its own definitions. If the law explicitly refers to some outside text, or if a court can construe the law to have been drafted with some outside text or an accepted common-law definition in mind, the court will look to that outside text or common-law definition in construing the statute. It is up to the court to decide how far afield to look. It is probably fair to say that a court will not invalidate a statute for vagueness unless it finds the statute morally repugnant and cannot come up with an alternate ground of unconstitutionality.[78]

All quoted phrases in the following paragraph are subject to attack, probably unsuccessful.

Under the PSRO law, sanctions can be imposed on physicians if they seek to obligate the federal government to pay for care which is not "medically necessary" and is not "of a quality which meets professionally recognized standards," when they fail to provide "evidence of such medical necessity and quality in such form and fashion and at such time as may reasonably be required" by the PSRO, or when they authorize a patient to be admitted to, or remain in, a hospital or other health facility when the patient's care can "consistent[ly] with professionally recognized . . . standards," be provided more cheaply in a different facility. Even so, sanctions can be imposed only when the physician has violated one or more of those obligations "in a substantial number" of cases, or "grossly and flagrantly" committed such violation one or more times.

"Gross" and "flagrant" are words which can be defined by the common law; "substantial number of cases" need not be defined in the statute because §1160(b) (1) implies that HEW has the right to determine how many violations must occur for the number to be considered "substantial" enough to trigger HEW's response. The terms "medically necessary" and "quality which meets professionally recognized standards" are both extremely vague, but the vagueness may be cured under two lines of argument. The common law, in cases of alleged malpractice, has developed a legally satisfactory evidentiary procedure for determining what are the "professionally recognized standards" in question; and the PSRO statute provides that the PSRO shall publish the criteria by which it will judge care. Therefore, even if the statute and regulations do not themselves define the "professionally recognized standards," a physician who is being judged will know, because of prior publication, what the standards are that he is being judged against.

It would be almost impossible to make a successful argument that either fifth amendment due process rights or sixth amendment rights to prior notification were violated by a statute or regulation which provided for such procedures. It would be a different legal case entirely if a PSRO chose to apply a sanction without first either publishing the criteria it intended to use or at least giving the sanctioned physician enough prior notice so that he had an opportunity to amend his practice. Assuming for the sake of argument that PSROs are at least quasi-governmental, and can therefore be sued for violating the constitutional rights of the parties subject to review, failure to specify the criteria or standards being used in judgment would itself probably be unconstitutional.

Improper Delegation

Can the federal government delegate its regulatory power to private agencies? The answer appears to be an unequivocal yes. Can it delegate that power when the private agency may be biased? The answer is, apparently, "no."

Delegation in General

For many years, the Supreme Court struggled with the problem of regulatory agencies. Those used to the modern idea that regulation is largely an executive function may be surprised that the Supreme Court's early cases established that regulation is, at least partially, a legislative power. The setting of standards against which conduct will be judged and unsatisfactory behavior punished is, in fact, an ultimate legislative power, and is therefore reserved to Congress by the Constitution.[79] The Supreme Court has nevertheless been able to justify executive agencies' rulemaking in an overwhelming number of cases.

The 1903 case of *Butterfield v. Stranahan*[80] illustrates an early method of resolving the problem. In that case, the Secretary of the Treasury was attacked for promulgating and using, as required by statute, a detailed set of quality standards for admitting or rejecting the importation of tea. The Supreme Court upheld both the Treasury's standards (as the question of their rationality had not been argued and was not subject to review) and its refusal of permission to import, saying, in part:

> We are of the opinion that the statute ... fixed a primary standard, and devolved upon the Secretary of the Treasury the mere executive duty to effectuate the legislative policy declared in the statute ... Congress legislated on the subject so far as was reasonably practicable. ...[81]

The "standard" enunciated in the act was that the tea not be "of inferior purity, quality, and fitness for consumption."[82] It must be noted, in fairness to the court and the Treasury Department, that an earlier act which remained in force and was, in effect, incorporated into the statute, did include a less general definition of what constituted "unfit" tea.[83] Despite the decision's restrictive language, it is apparent that even at the turn of the century the Supreme Court was giving executive agencies broad rulemaking powers.

By the time of the New Deal and the start of the explosive growth of regulatory agencies, the Court's requirements had become more elaborate and routine. A good example of the Supreme Court's depression-era position is the landmark case of *Schechter Poultry Corp. v. U.S.*,[84] in which the Court, in striking down the National Industrial Recovery Act, discussed, in dicta, the conditions without which it would invalidate as unconstitutional any regulatory agency's authority. These conditions included: (1) statutory limitation of executive power,[85] (2) provisions for notice and hearing for those affected by the regulatory process,[86] (3) a requirement that executive action be taken only after evidence had been collected and findings of fact made[87] to justify any contemplated regulatory action.

The Court's requirements and Congress's instructions for carrying them out were eventually codified as the Administrative Procedures Act (APA) in 1946. The Act does not cover all agencies nor all the activities of any agency, but it does cover most, including rulemaking and adjudication. While it is possible to constitutionally delegate rulemaking or adjudicatory authority to a group not covered by the APA, Congress can usually be assured of a court finding of constitutionality whenever it delegates authority to an agency covered by the APA or whose rules are substantially identical.

In this context, it should be obvious that delegation to a nongovernmental entity will ordinarily be found constitutional as long as that group, organization, or person observes due process in carrying out its delegated functions. In case there is any doubt, however, a number of Supreme Court cases have held explicitly that such delegation is proper. For example, in *St. Louis & Iron Mt. Ry. v. Taylor*,[88] a 1907 case, the Court upheld a rulemaking procedure affecting the height of "draw bars" on railway freight cars where the standard had been written by the American Railway Association and adopted verbatim by the Interstate Commerce Commission. More modern cases exist, of course, but the legal principle remains constant.

The Question of Bias

One of the few occasions in which a court will declare unconstitutional a delegation to a group covered by APA or its equivalent is when the court finds an unavoidable bias or self-interest, no matter how correct the group's procedures. The rule that those subject to regulation should not be forced to abide by decisions which are tainted by bias or self-interest will also invalidate specific decisions made on an impermissible basis by members of an agency or group permitted delegation.

Although fairness and good faith will ordinarily be presumed, that presumption can be overcome by evidence of actual bias or self-interest. For example, in *Gibson v. Berryhill*,[89] a 1973 case, the U.S. Supreme Court said that it was proper for a lower court to set aside a ruling by the Alabama Board of Optometry, a group normally presumed able to exercise its delegated functions, when there was clear evidence that the ruling in question had been tainted by self-interest. The Alabama Board had been prohibited by law from choosing members who were not members of the state's optometrists' association, which in turn had bylaws admitting to membership only self-employed optometrists. The Board ruled that an Alabama statute, which had been amended to remove optometric offices from department stores and similar nonmedical establishments, should be interpreted as prohibiting the practice of optometry by anyone not self-employed. When a group of optometrists who worked for a branch of an optometric chain found themselves subject to licensure revocation proceedings, they sued. The Supreme Court, noting that the members of the Alabama Board would have found themselves the beneficiaries of the customer shift which would have occurred if their disciplinary proceedings had been allowed to run to completion, held that it was not improper for the federal District Court to move to stop the Board before it could take final action.

Delegation and the PSRO Program

How does the law on delegation and bias apply to the PSRO program? Briefly, it appears that congressional delegation of both rulemaking and adjudicatory authority to the PSROs is, on its face, fully constitutional. That the PSROs may be "private" corporations rather than "governmental" agencies—a matter which we do not believe has been legally settled—is immaterial: public or private, PSROs can indeed exercise the authority they have been given by the statute. The only two things which could potentially block PSRO operations, in the context of a delegation argument, would be a court's finding of an absence of due process in PSRO activities or of bias in PSRO decision-making.

A finding of lack of due process in the PSRO statute is unlikely in the extreme, as there is nothing in the statute which would preclude the most stringent imaginable due-process regulations from being drafted by HEW for the PSROs.[90] A finding of lack of due process in specific regulations is considerably more likely. To take one example: there are, as yet, no specific regulations on the publication of treatment criteria. If a physician, group of physicians, hospital, nursing home, or other affected person, institution, or association were to attack a PSRO's criteria-setting procedures on the grounds, inter alia, that the criteria were not published early enough or distributed widely enough to permit sufficient input from those affected, a court could easily find either: (1) that the regulations governing that aspect of PSRO operations were insufficiently stringent, entirely absent, or too vague and must therefore be discarded and replaced by legally and constitutionally adequate regulations; or (2) that the PSRO's procedure was itself constitutionally inadequate, regardless of the status of HEW's regulations, and that the plaintiff physician and others similarly situated, and the payor agencies, should not consider themselves bound by those criteria until correct procedures were observed by the defendant PSRO.

If the court were to decide in the course of such a lawsuit that PSROs were federal agencies and, as such, had to publish their criteria in the *Federal Register,* that would not change the issues in the case nor necessarily affect the outcome. Due process is due process,[91] at least in its essential features, and any delegated group, PSROs included, has to observe at least some of the formalities.

A finding of bias or self-interest in PSRO operations is unlikely, although, as was argued in Chapter 3, the possibility of a "cost-cutting" bias, resulting from PSROs' interest in self-preservation, may well exist. Two things which will save the program and the PSROs from adverse court decisions on this question are: (1) the permissible nature of the "bias" and (2) the legal presumption in favor of good faith.

Briefly, the worst thing that can be said about any HEW or PSRO tendency to reduce Medicare/Medicaid reimbursement in any given instance is that such a tendency is exactly what the PSRO statute appears to demand.[92] That PSRO review boards may find themselves tempted to judge physicians and hospitals "guilty" until proven innocent, once payment denial has been recommended, will probably not be regarded by the courts as a constitutionally impermissible bias. Furthermore, the legal presumption that fairness and good faith will obtain in PSRO and HEW adjudications may have a firm factual basis. And unless facts can be established with sufficient force to overcome the presumption, the PSROs are safe.

One must note, however, that a possibility of real bias always exists in any regulatory scheme which permits peers to judge peers. If a "swing-vote" member of a PSRO review board were to make a decision against a fellow physician on the basis of, for example, a personal vendetta, and the victimized physician could prove that hatred or envy, rather than reasoned judgment, was the basis for payment denial or other disciplinary action, no court would allow the PSRO's decision to stand. Of course, the plaintiff physician would have to prove not only that the bias existed, but that it made a difference or at least could have had a sufficient influence to taint the entire proceeding.

CONCLUSION

Is the PSRO program constitutional? At this time the answer seems to be: probably. While it appears that PSRO review will in some sense restrict patients and physicians in their exercise of their rights to privacy in the treatment relationship, and will impinge on physicians' right to practice their profession, the best argument appears to be that such infringements are probably not repugnant to the Constitution. Furthermore, the statute appears to be neither so broadly drafted nor so vague that it violates the fifth amendment. Nevertheless, if a litigant opposing the PSRO program were able to prove to a court's satisfaction that the review process resulted in harm to an already disadvantaged group of patients, or that the immediate effects of review included a potential or actual deprivation of the right to life of any patient, the possibility of an anti-PSRO decision would be increased. Ultimately, in short, the decision about the program's constitutionality turns more on questions of fact than on questions of law, important as the legal questions will be in guiding the courts in deciding which facts are important. And that, quite possibly, is as it should be: if the program does harm, it should be abolished or modified; and if it does not do harm and carries potential for benefit, it should be given a chance.

NOTES

1. 395 F. Supp 125 (1975). [hereinafter AAPS].

2. D.C. N.D. E.D. Ill. Docket No. 75-C-560 [hereinafter AMA hearing]; 522 F.2d 921 (1975) [hereinafter AMA appeal].

3. The brief has been published as part of Appendix H to the transcript of the Hearings on Implementation of PSRO Legislation [PL 92-603] before the Subcommittee on Health of the Senate Committee on Finance, 93rd Cong., 2nd Sess., pts. 1 & 2 (1974) [hereinafter 1974 Hearings].

4. The groups may be referred to as: (1) professional practice, (2) physician-patient relationship, (3) privacy, (4) vagueness and uncertainty, (5) liability limit in §1167, (6) licensure, and (7) delegation of quasi-judicial authority. The government made two "affirmative defenses:" that the court lacked jurisdiction and that the PSRO law was "a valid exercise of Congressional power." 1974 Hearings at 944.

5. The court's grouping paralleled the government's with the addition of a "section (8)"

on the alleged inefficiency and lack of necessity for the program. The court, however, characterized the AAPS's case as having seven grounds.

6. AAPS at 132.

7. AAPS at 139. In all fairness to the AAPS, it should be pointed out that this language reflects the Supreme Court's position in the 1973 abortion cases, infra. While it is impossible to predict how far those cases can be stretched, they do contain at least a suggestion that some licensure rights are so basic that they cannot be removed even after due process. Whether the Supreme Court would accept such a reading is highly doubtful.

8. Plaintiffs' Complaint at 12, AAPS; 1974 Hearings at 880.

9. §1156(a), 42 USC 1320c-5(a).

10. Doe v. Bolton, 410 U.S. 179 (1973) [hereinafter Doe]; Roe v. Wade, 410 U.S. 113 (1973) [hereinafter Roe].

11. AAPS at 136.

12. Id.

13. Id. at 137.

14. Id.

15. *See, e.g.*, California Bankers Assn. v. Shultz, 416 U.S. 21 (1974). Obviously, prior cases can be distinguished on their facts. A discussion of related problems can be found in Chapter 6.

16. AAPS at 140.

17. Id. at 131.

18. Id. at 132.

19. Id. at 133.

20. Id. at 134.

21. Id.

22. Id. at 132.

23. Id. at 133.

24. Id. at 134.

25. Id. at 141.

26. Id.

27. Id. at 138.

28. Id.

29. Id. at 133.

30. Id. at 140.

31. Id.

32. Plaintiffs' Complaint at 8, AMA hearing.

33. Id.

34. Plaintiffs' Memo at 6, AMA hearing.

35. Doe. supra, note 10.

36. 381 U.S. 479 (1965).

37. Plaintiffs' Memo at 7, AMA hearing.

38. Id. at 9.

39. Id. at 14.

40. Id. at 15. The Medicare Hospital Manual (HIM 10) §290, by denying reimbursement, effectively prohibits nontotal review.

41. AMA hearing at 20.

42. Transcript May 27, 1975, at 9, AMA hearing: "the court . . . is not . . . impressed by the arguments of the physician plaintiffs that contrary findings by review committees will irreparably damage their professional reputations or expose them to malpractice actions. . . ."

43. AMA hearing at 15.

44. Id. at 16.

45. Id. at 21.

46. AMA appeal at 4, 10. The "as presented" language refers to the appellate court's statement that some government evidence had been improperly excluded at the hearing.

47. AMA hearing at 19.

48. A statute will be declared unconstitutional if it is so vague that any attempt to enforce it would interfere with fifth-amendment due-process rights; overbreadth may be repugnant to many different parts of the Constitution. We are treating the issues separately primarily to increase the clarity of the discussion.

49. Certain issues, while crucial to any litigation which might actually be brought, are not relevant to the abstract questions of constitutionality. For example, the question of ripeness would not be raised if the plaintiffs were to wait until a sanction (such as nonpayment) had been imposed on them by a PSRO and appealed through the PSRO process; on the other hand, when a suit is brought between the issuance of the regulations and the imposition of the first sanction, the question of ripeness would have to be argued. (Although plaintiffs must ordinarily wait for a harm to occur before a suit is considered ripe, it is generally accepted that one need not wait to become the victim of adverse official action if one can argue that the regulations under which the action is about to be taken are unavoidably and irremediably harmful.)

Similarly, the question of standing need not be an overwhelming problem. Although the Supreme Court held in Tileston v. Ullman, 318 U.S. 44 (1973), that a physician cannot assert a claim for a patient's right to treatment; nothing prevents patients or potential patients from joining the plaintiff's cause; and physicians of course have standing to assert a claim of their own (e.g., right to practice one's profession). In general, federal courts have not been anxious to dispose of "right to treatment" cases on the grounds of lack of standing, unripeness, mootness, etc., in recent years. Compare, e.g., Doe or Roe, with Poe v. Ullman, 367 U.S. 497 (1961).

50. Doe, supra, note 10.

51. Roe, supra, note 10.

52. Roe at 153.

53. Doe at 197.

54. Roe at 152.

55. What the court did in the abortion decisions was to adopt a "sliding scale" of compulsion; the state's interest was said to become increasingly compelling as the fetus neared term. There was, therefore, no overall decision on the question. See Roe at 156.

56. Doe at 197.

57. Roe at 154.

58. The Court referred to *Jacobson v. Mass.* (197 U.S. 11 (1905)), on vaccination, and *Buck v. Bell* (274 U.S. 200 (1927)), on compulsory sterilization. At least the Buck decision

has been somewhat restricted by *Skinner v. Oklahoma* (316 U.S. 535 (1942)), which limits the state's power by applying strict due process standards.

59. Roe at 154.

60. There are differences, of course. For example, the Georgia law provided that physicians who successfully performed illegal abortions could be jailed for up to ten years. The physician who breaks the PSRO law is subject only to a fine (unless he or she wrongfully releases confidential data while acting as the PSRO's agent or employee). In general, the more severe the punishment, the more carefully the law will be scrutinized.

61. Doe at 195.

62. Id. at 199.

63. Id. at 199.

64. See, e.g., McLaughlin v. Florida, 379 U.S. 184 (1964); Bolling v. Sharpe, 347 U.S. 497, 499 (1954); Korematsu v. U.S., 323 U.S. 214, 216, 223 (1944); Virginia Bd. of Elections v. Hamm, 230 F. Supp. 156 (1964), aff'd 379 U.S. 19 (1964).

65. See, e.g., Frontiero v. Richardson, 411 U.S. 677, 682, 688 (1971); Reed v. Reed, 404 U.S. 71 (1971); but see, contra, Frontiero at 691, 692; Kahn v. Shevin, 416 U.S. 351 (1974).

66. See, e.g., Harper v. Virginia Bd. of Elections, 383 U.S. 663, 668 (1968); McDonald v. Bd. of Election Commissioners, 394 U.S. 802, 807 (1969). U.S. Dept. Ag. v. Moreno, 413 U.S. 528 (1973), invalidating an anti-"hippie" provision in the food stamp law, is related.

67. Analogies could, perhaps, be made to the *de facto* segregation cases.

68. Roe at 192.

69. Forgotson, Cook, "Innovations and Experiments in the Use of Health Manpower—the Effect of Licensure Laws," 32 *Law and Contemporary Problems* 561 (1967).

70. See, e.g., Doe at 188, 189.

71. Griswold.

72. As well as other constitutional protections. See, e.g., Geduldig v. Aiello, 417 U.S. 424 (1974); VonStauffenberg v. Unemployment Compensation Bd., 459 F.2d 1128, 1130 (1972) at 1130 (equal protection). As the *Geduldig* majority stated, "Particularly with respect to social welfare programs, so long as the line drawn by the state is nationally supportable, the courts will not interpose their judgment as to the appropriate stopping point." Opinion at 495.

73. U.S. Const. amend. V.

74. Fleming v. Nestor, 363 U.S. 603 (1960).

75. 73 Yale L. J. 733 (1964).

76. See, e.g., Goldberg v. Kelly, 397 U.S. 254, 264 (1970); Wheeler v. Montgomery, 397 U.S. 280 (1970).

77. There is no evidence that Congress or HEW compared a retrospective-plus-limited-nonretrospective screening procedure to a concurrent-plus-other-nonretrospective screening procedure performed by roughly equivalent groups upon roughly equivalent patient and provider populations to determine whether or not the statute's bias in favor of the more invasive (and expensive) forms of review is justified. In fact, the most that Congress was able to say, at the time the law was passed, was that purely retrospective claims review was inferior to purely concurrent utilization review in the Medicare and Medicaid Programs.

78. An example of this can be seen in the debate over the Washington, D.C., antiabortion law in the 1972 decision U.S. v. Vuitch (402 US 62). One of the questions in the case was

whether or not the word "health" was unconstitutionally vague. The majority held that the word "health" could only be interpreted by a reasonable man as "soundness of body or mind," and was therefore not vague. Justice Douglas, in dissent, wrote that if the statute left the definition of "health" to the physician, without defining the type or degree of disease or risk required to constitute a threat sufficient to justify an abortion on "protection of health" grounds, it must therefore follow that the accuracy of the physician's interpretation was a jury question, and this would require the physician to second-guess the community's moral standard every time he did a procedure; Justice Douglas found this to be impermissible. Justice Stewart, also in dissent, argued to the contrary that the statute, by not defining "health," compelled a reading that the physician's definition was binding on all parties, and that prosecution for violation was therefore impossible; this reading would have upheld the statute at the cost of its enforceability. The various justices' decisions as to whether the statute was impermissibly vague or not depended on whether they wished to invalidate it, and, if so, how.

79. U.S. Const. art. I, §8.

80. 192 U.S. 470 (1903).

81. Id. at 496.

82. Id. at 472. It is remarkable how closely this language resembles that of the PSRO statute.

83. Id. at 495.

84. 295 U.S. 495 (1935).

85. Id. at 538.

86. Id. at 539.

87. Id. at 538, 540.

88. 210 U.S. 281, 286, 287 (1908).

89. 411 U.S. 564 (1973).

90. It should be noted that congressional intent was probably to exempt PSROs from some of the due process requirements which govern HEW itself (see Chapter 5, *infra.*). However, congressional intent is not binding, and the courts will save the statute, and the program, if they have to, by ignoring congressional intent and looking only at the statutory language. Unconstitutionality will not be presumed.

91. Obviously, we are ignoring the fine distinctions here. There are variations in the rules of evidence, formality of notification, etc.

92. §1151, 42 USC 1320c; see, for a physician-lawyer's interpretation, M. Segal, "A Hard Look at the PSRO Law," *J. Legal Med.* 2 (Oct. 1974): 16, "Reading the legislation, one sees the word 'cost' and then the words 'and quality control,' but if one eliminated 'and quality control' at every single point . . . this law would operate exactly the same."

Chapter 5

Are PSROs Federal
Agencies?

In §1152(b)(1) of the PSRO statute, Professional Standards Review Organizations are defined as nonprofit professional associations, although the Secretary may designate a public corporation or agency as a PSRO. It is the official policy of HEW that PSROs are to be classified as private organizations, incorporated under the state laws of their respective jurisdictions. By and large, for purposes of this text, it has been irrelevant whether or not PSROs were nonprofit corporations. In examining the structure and functions of PSROs, however, it becomes apparent that these organizations are unique in that they do not conform to the structure of most private corporations. It is our contention, moreover, that the severe constraints placed upon the PSRO by HEW far exceed the types of controls to which federal contractors are generally subject.

It is the function of this chapter to present a number of the reasons why the authors believe that the PSRO may, in fact, be considered a type of federal agency. PSROs' agency status will be evaluated primarily with respect to two pieces of federal legislation: the Federal Tort Claims Act and the Freedom of Information Act. One should note that although a PSRO may be considered an agency in various situations under certain pieces of legislation, it does not necessarily have general agency status for all purposes.[1]

BACKGROUND

PSROs, like other federal contractors, are subject to the requirements of the Federal Procurement Manual and the monitoring of a project and a contract officer. Unlike other federal contractors, PSROs must comply

119

with a greater than usual number of constraints, covering all phases of PSRO operations. The Bureau of Quality Assurance (BQA) has managed the PSRO program by use of policy guidelines (transmittal letters, policy statements, PSRO manuals) which technically are designed to serve as a source of guidance, but in most cases have been implemented as though they were regulations.[2]

The regulations to be issued by HEW in running the PSRO program will constitute control over almost all aspects of PSRO organization and review. The present transmittal letters alone demonstrate the extensiveness of BQA requirements. There is no question that PSROs in their start-up phase need federal assistance, but there is a difference between assistance and control. The actions of BQA go beyond being advisory. PSROs are placed in a paradoxical situation: Federal policy indicates that they are to be private, independent entities, yet they are able to act only as specified in BQA guidelines, and they must await those guidelines before they can take action.

In assessing the PSRO's status as a type of federal agency, the issue of control is not the only important factor. In conducting medical review to determine the appropriateness, necessity and quality of health care services for Titles XVIII, XIX, and V patients, the PSROs have the legal authority to render final determinations as to whether patients should be hospitalized. In making such a determination the PSRO is making a "governmental decision," the PSRO does not merely assist HEW (as other contractors may), but it possesses binding powers that are akin to the type of authority possessed by an agency.

PSROs do have the option, if they desire, to conduct review activities for private parties, such as Blue Cross or some other commercial carrier. In fact, PSROs may be forced for their own survival to seek alternative funding sources in the private sector. However, the fact that PSROs engage in private review does not alter the argument that these entities may be federal agencies for certain purposes. It is our contention that the PSRO is acting as a federal agency when it conducts medical review for Titles XVII, XIX, and V patients.

COMPARISONS

While a number of useful analogies can be drawn between PSROs and government entities such as public authorities or public corporations, these comparisons are not dispositive.

One could compare a nonprofit corporation created under law for public purposes, such as Amtrak (National Railroad Passenger Corporation Act),[3] with a PSRO. While Amtrak was established specifically as a private corporation, as were PSROs, it is often classified as a public entity. As was commented in *Business Law*: "There are numerous indications throughout the act (National Railroad Passenger Corporation Act) and in the composition of its Board of Directors that Amtrak's public nature is intended to be dominant . . . the dominance of Amtrak's public attributes makes it difficult to resist the conclusion that, although ostensibly a private public utility, Amtrak is for all intents and purposes an instrument of national policy."[4] It seems reasonable that if legal commentators view Amtrak as a public entity, one could argue that a PSRO, with far less flexibility in its operational sphere and an equally high degree of accountability, is also a public entity.

On the surface, when one compares organizational and operating structures, the similarities can be minimized between a public corporation like Amtrak and a PSRO. The fact is, however, PSROs and public corporations are not fundamentally very different, for they are legislatively created, publically funded entities, performing functions that are governmental in nature. PSROs, if anything, have a stronger tie to the government than do most public corporations. Still, there is no question that the comparison between PSROs and public corporations is difficult because there is no precedent for PSRO. It would seem that legal commentators, and eventually the courts, who have tended to look beyond the private structure of Amtrak in finding a public entity, would not hesitate to do likewise in the case of PSROs.

PSRO: AGENCY UNDER FEDERAL LAW

While it may be an interesting exercise to evaluate the PSRO's legal status, it is most useful when such concern is related to some specific area of federal legislation. Even if PSROs are not agents or agencies of the federal government for all purposes, they may qualify for such status under certain specific federal laws. For example, for purposes of the Freedom of Information Act[5] PSROs could be classified as agencies, even if they are not so classified for purposes of other federal acts. HEW's current policy is that PSROs are private corporations and never fall within the definition of agency; this position is adopted for purposes of consistency, but the policy may not be defensible in all cases. Some federal courts may look to the unique public purpose of PSROs, and hold that certain federal enactments are applicable to these structures.

Among the more significant legislation that may apply to PSROs are the Freedom of Information Act, the Privacy Act, the Civil Rights Act of

1964, the Administrative Procedures Act, and the Federal Tort Claims Act.[6] It is not our intent to review all of these statutes to determine their potential applicability to PSRO, but rather to use the Federal Tort Claims Act, the Freedom of Information Act, and, briefly, the Administrative Procedures Act as examples of laws which cause us to argue that PSROs act as agencies of the federal government.

Federal Tort Claims Act

The Federal Tort Claims Act (FTCA),[7] passed in the 1940's, abolished for the federal government in certain limited cases the doctrine of sovereign immunity. This doctrine prevents governmental instrumentalities from being held liable for the civil wrongs of their employees. The Act extends the doctrine of "respondeat superior" to persons employed by the federal government or those acting on behalf of a federal agency; that is, the act makes the government as an employer liable for the torts of an employee. The FTCA section that defines "agency" expressly excludes "any contractor with the U.S."[8] In fact, however, the section excluding government contractors is not all that clear, for there are instances when a contractor may lose his independent status and fall under the act.

In order to be classified as an independent contractor, an organization or individual must be able to exercise a degree of independence over the means, method, and manner of carrying out an agreed-upon task. If a federal contractor is forced to comply with federally imposed requirements so stringent that the contractor cannot function independently, then federal courts view the contractor as losing its independent status; and its employees would then fall within the scope of the FTCA. Federal courts have begun to look beyond the fact that an organization is under contract with the government and question whether a contractor is acting freely, or is being so severely restricted as to lose that ability.

In the case of *Schetter v. Housing Authority of the City of Erie*,[9] it was held that a public housing authority was actually a government instrumentality, even though the terms of a contract stated that the housing authority was an independent contractor. "It was pointed out that when a lease shrouds the relationship between the Government and an agency, courts should pierce the veil in order to avoid an evasion of the governmental responsibility. Considering the actualities of the relationship and noting the extent of control retained by the government, the court held that the defendant was in reality a managing agent for the U.S., rather than a lessee and, therefore, the Government was responsible."[10] Other cases involving federal contracts in the community housing area have also held that the contractor is acting on behalf of the federal government, and, therefore, the contractor's employees come within the terms of the FTCA. As a general rule, "In deciding whether a given relationship is that of principal and agent or principal and independent contractor, the courts are concerned primarily with the type and extent of control retained by the principal ... the greater the control, the greater is the likelihood of a finding of agency."[11]

In the case of *Orleans v. United States,*[12] the plaintiff brought suit against the Government to recover for injuries suffered in an automobile accident while riding in a car hired by the Warren Trumbell Council for Economic Opportunity, which was transporting children to a field day outing. The government answered the complaint by arguing that the W.T.C.E.O. was not an agent or instrumentality of the U.S. but a private nonprofit corporation, and that, therefore, the government could not be held liable under the Federal Tort Claims Act for the negligence which led to the accident. The regional OEO Director argued that the W.T.C.E.O. was a private corporation, conducted its own business under contract with the Office of Economic Opportunity, and, by and large, acted independently of government supervision.

A federal court of appeals disagreed with the government position and ruled that a Community Action Council, formed for purposes of the Economic Opportunity Act, receiving funds solely from the federal government and operating within statutory and regulatory OEO guidelines was, in fact, acting as a federal agency for purposes of the FTCA. The court of appeals felt that the powers the OEO held over the Community Action Council were "not powers usually possessed by a principal in dealing with an independent contractor."[13] The court used the issue of control as a barometer in determining whether a federal contractor was exercising sufficient independence to fall outside the Federal Tort Claims Act.

The Court of Appeals decision in the Orleans case was, however, overturned by the U.S. Supreme Court. The Court felt that Congress intended in the Economic Opportunity Act to establish local independent private entities that were to develop community action programs.[14] The fact that the community action organizations were funded by the government did not make them governmental agencies. The Court pointed out that if this were the case, the Federal Tort Claims Act would be expanded far beyond the intent of Congress "and cover countless unidentifiable classes of beneficiaries."[15] The Court felt that OEO regulations and guidelines were designed to assure that federal money be spent for the purposes of the program, not to control the operations of these local groups.

The Court did not really deal with the issue of control, which was so persuasive in the Court of Appeals' decisions. The Supreme Court merely evaluated the status of the local community action program as an entity under contract to the government, receiving funds and advice from OEO. Such analysis ignored the extent of control OEO exercised over the community action programs; for while theoretically these local organizations could operate independently, actually they were tightly controlled by federal regulations.

The fact that the Supreme Court reached the conclusion in the Orleans case that the Federal Tort Claims Act did not apply to community action organizations does not necessarily mean that the FTCA will not apply to PSROs. A court's view of the facts in a case is often dependent on the outcome desired. If a court wishes to reach the conclusion that a PSRO is a federal agency, it will look at the extent of control BQA has exercised over individual PSROs and the fact that the government is dictating all major PSRO financial and operational policies. If the judiciary wishes to avoid application of the Federal Tort Claims Act to PSROs, the courts will avoid using the test of control in evaluating their legal status. In such a case the court would follow the Supreme Court rationale in the Orleans case, looking at the PSRO statute and official HEW policy alone, without assessing the realities of how PSROs function. If, however, the control test is used, there is a strong chance that PSROs would be held to fall under the Federal Tort Claims Act and that the government would therefore be responsible for indemnifying those injured by a PSRO employee.[16]

Freedom of Information Act

The Federal Freedom of Information Act (FOIA), as discussed earlier in this chapter, requires each federal agency to make information it holds available to the public in accordance with published rules, provided such data is not exempt under the terms of the Act. The 1974 amendments to the Freedom of Information Act expanded the definitions of "agency" to include "executive departments, military departments, government corporations, government-controlled corporations, and independent regulatory agencies."[17] The trend continues to be to widen the scope of FOIA application.

Whether an entity will come within the terms of the FOIA depends upon an individual judicial determination. In view of the expanding scope of the agency concept for purposes of the Act, an argument can be made for including PSROs within this statute. Presently, only PSRO data that is directly reported to HEW falls under the FOIA. But if the

Act is applicable to the local organizations, all data, including that which is personally identifiable, may be accessible.*[18]

Since the "agency" definition in the amended Freedom of Information Act has not yet been interpreted, we can only speculate on how broadly it should be construed. It could be argued that a PSRO, similar to Amtrak or the Corporation for Public Broadcasting, is a corporate entity; while not owned by the government, is, indeed, under tight federal control, having little flexibility of operation, and as such comes under the FOIA definition of agency. Our interpretation is dependent on the way in which we evaluate the legislative history of the amended FOIA statute, for the House Report on the amendment upholds the position that corporations not federally owned but federally controlled fall within the agency definition.[19] The conference committee report states that the conferees "do not intend to include corporations which receive appropriated funds but are neither chartered by the Federal Government nor controlled by it."**[20]

Because PSROs are chartered by the states but controlled by the federal government, in order to determine whether they can be classified as agencies under the Freedom of Information Act, we must seek an answer outside the statutory language or legislative history. A number of court decisions bearing directly on the agency question may help in evaluating the PSROs' status. In the case of *Soucie v. David**[21] the court determined that the Office of Science and Technology was an agency for purposes of the Administrative Procedures Act, based on the rationale that any administrative unit with substantial independent authority in specific functions has agency status.[22] In *Washington Research Proj. Inc. v. Dept. of H.E.W.*,[23] the court decided that the initial project review groups for the National Advisory Mental Health Council were not federal agencies because they acted only in an advisory capacity without authority to make final decisions. The court in the Washington Research Project case felt that the question of determining agency status rested upon "whether an entity has any authority in law to make decisions."[24]

In *Renegotiation Board v. Grumman Aircraft Eng. Corp.*,[25] the court found that a regional renegotiation board was a federal agency for pur-

---

*Of course this access may be barred by the exemption provisions discussed in the Confidentiality chapter.

**The Freedom of Information Act is a part of the Administrative Procedures Act (APA) (Title V of the U.S. Code). Therefore, arguments about agency status under the APA can be applied to the FOIA. It is also possible to argue that if PSROs fall within the scope of the new agency provisions in the Freedom of Information Act, the Administrative Procedures Act is applicable to PSROs. Extension of the APA to PSROs would mean that these corporate bodies have to follow federal rule-making procedure in developing policy.

poses of the Freedom of Information Act. The court in this case cited a study by Professor James O. Freedman, whose analysis of what constituted an agency was based upon a determination of where the administrative power to act rested. The court case concluded that the Regional Boards in question were agencies because they served as a "discrete, decision-making layer" in the contract renegotiation process. The United States Supreme Court, in reviewing the *Renegotiation Board v. Grumman Aircraft* case (and overturning it on other grounds), did not discuss the agency question, but in a footnote indicated its agreement with the lower court's position. The Supreme Court noted that the regional board in question had power to issue orders only in a certain kind of case; therefore, its status as an agency would be limited to matters in this specific class of cases, somewhat narrowing the scope of the agency definition. In the case of *Wolfe v. Weinberger*[26] the court ruled that an advisory review panel, which was appointed to receive and evaluate information on antacids, and which submitted a report to the commissioner of FDA but had no authority in law to make decisions, was not an "agency" within the terms of the Freedom of Information Act. It is interesting to note that while the advisory committee in question was not considered within the FOIA agency definition, it comes within the bounds of the Federal Advisory Committee Act,[27] which allows public access to their deliberations.

Case law demonstrates that the primary issue in determining whether a given entity is an "agency" for purposes of the Freedom of Information Act is whether that entity has legal authority to make decisions. The PSRO statute empowers PSROs to make decisions in medical review, denial of payment, sanction and appeal, etc. (§1155, 1158, 1160). Indeed, in the area of medical review, a PSRO has the legal authority to make final determinations about the quality, necessity and appropriateness of services delivered under Titles XVIII, XIX, and V. The PSROs then advise HEW in the operation of Medicare, Medicaid, and the Maternal and Child Health programs and they do not merely function as advisory groups to the Secretary. Certainly the authority of PSROs to make final determinations, coupled with the expanded agency definition which the Congressional conference committee applied to government-controlled but not owned corporations, indicate that PSROs could fall within the act's agency definition.

Administrative Procedures Act

The Administrative Procedures Act[28] (APA) passed in 1946 serves as the basis for federal agency procedures to ensure uniformity of agency operations. Until recently, it would have been difficult to argue that the APA could be applied to PSROs, since the original agency definition in this act was rather narrow. In 1974, however, the agency definition was broadened, as discussed previously,[29] in the amendments to the Freedom of Information Act, which is part of the APA. It follows that this same agency definition would make the Administrative Procedures Act applicable to PSROs.

The ramifications of applying the APA to PSROs may be felt in two areas (treating the FOIA as a distinct and separate area): adjudicatory procedures and rulemaking. But even in these areas, the effect may be superficial at best. The current BQA policies for PSRO adjudicatory functions are such that application of the APA in this area would not radically change current procedures. The PSRO structure as it is developing in the hearing and appeals area is sufficient to fulfill the APA's adjudicatory requirements and thus in this area only minor alterations may be required. Application of the rulemaking process to PSROs would mean that an individual PSRO would have to issue guidelines or policy directives through the *Federal Register*. The actual rulemaking, however, would still be a function of HEW, as policy for PSROs is generally made on a national and not local level. So it would seem that the application of APA rulemaking clauses to individual PSROs would have little impact on local operations, other than an infrequent inconvenience.

CONCLUSION

There has been an attempt by the Bureau of Quality Assurance to comply with the spirit of several major pieces of federal legislation (e.g., Privacy Act, Civil Rights Act of 1964) without expressly holding that the PSRO falls within their bounds. As a result, HEW has developed parallel policies similar to major pieces of federal legislation for the PSRO. An example can be demonstrated in the confidentiality area, where the PSRO guidelines closely resemble the Privacy Act. To conform to its policy that the PSRO is to be treated as an independent government contractor, HEW consistently holds that the PSRO is not, for any purpose, a federal agency.

If the PSRO is classified as a federal agency for certain purposes (for example, the Federal Tort Claims Act), this classification may eventually be extended into other areas, and HEW's characterization of such bodies may be lost. It seems that HEW wants PSROs to remain private entities both to avoid the constraints of federal law and to ensure the support of local physician groups. There is no doubt that if the medical community views the PSRO as a federal agency, their resistance may become even stronger.[30]

While implementing the PSRO program as a federal agency may pose certain practical, legal, and organizational barriers, to hold the position that the PSRO is strictly a private nonprofit corporation, merely contracting with the federal government, constitutes irresponsible policy.

HEW is attempting to govern by contract, using PSROs to carry out what are clearly federal agency functions. PSROs may be more manageable and politically acceptable as independent private contractors, but as entities carrying out a public function, they should have the same degree of accountability and protection under federal law as other agencies. By treating the PSRO solely as a federal contractor, HEW is not only denying the reality of the strict limitations placed on the operation of a PSRO organization by the federal government, it is also denying the public certain constitutional and regulatory protections afforded under federal law.

NOTES

1. Freedam, James O., "Administrative Procedure and the Control of Foreign Direct Investment," 119 *U. Pa. Law Review* 6–9 (1970).

2. DHEW, *PSRO Manual* (Washington: BQA 1974, 75, 76). See Also *PSRO Transmittal Letters,* No. 1–41.

3. National Railroad Corporation Act, 45 USC §541.

4. Adams, Arnold, "The National Railroad Passenger Corporation—A Modern Hybrid Corporation," 31 *Business Law* 601 (1976).

5. Federal Freedom of Information Act 5 USC §552(3) (Supp. Feb. 1975).

6. Federal Tort Claims Act, 28 USC §1346(b) & 2671 et seq.

7. Id.

8. Id.

9. Schetter v. Housing Authority of the City of Erie, 132 F. Supp. 149 (W.D. Pa. 1955).

10. Id.

11. Id.

12. Orleans v. United States, 44 L.W. 4703 (1976).

13. Id.

14. Id.
"Nothing could be plainer than the Congressional intent that the local entities here in question have complete control over operations of their own program with the federal government providing financial aid, advice and oversight. . . ."

15. Id.

16. *Supra* at note 6, §2671, see Orleans v. U.S., 509 F.2d 197 (1975).
If the Federal Tort Claims Act applies to the PSRO, the immunity provision in the PSRO law would not be nearly as important to individuals working for the organization. Even if an individual acting on behalf of PSROs failed to exercise due care, he would be covered

from liability by virtue of the FTCA. The ramifications for the government would be more serious, for application of this Act would mean indemnification for employee torts.

17. 5 USC §552(3) (Supp. Feb. 1975).

18. Access under the federal Freedom of Information Act may be barred by virtue of the exemption provisions discussed in Chapter 6.

19. H.R. 93-876. See, "Definition of Agency."

20. H.R. 93-1380, Conference Report, "Expansion of the Agency Definition."

21. Soucie v. David, 448 F.2d 1067 (1971).

22. Id.

23. Washington Research Project v. DHEW, 504 F.2d 2318 (1974).

24. Id.

25. Renegotiation Board v. Gruman Aircraft, 482 F.2d 710 (D.C. Cir. 1974).

26. Wolfe v. Weinberger, 403 F. Supp. 238 (1975).

27. Federal Advisory Committee Act, 5 USC §10(b) appendix.

28. Administrative Procedures Act, 5 USC §1001-1011.

29. FOIA, *supra,* at note 17.

30. See Chapter 3, Provider Concerns.

Chapter 6

Confidentiality and Peer Review

The PSRO, in carrying out its review functions, will collect, generate and store massive amounts of data on practitioners, providers and patients. Much of the data collected by a peer review organization will be somewhat routine, but a significant portion of it will deal with sensitive issues involving patients, physicians and institutions. There is great concern about how PSROs will handle sensitive data. Questions about what PSRO information will be protected and how those protections will be implemented are major areas of debate influenced by a developing body of law dealing with the individual's privacy rights.

While the Bureau of Quality Assurance has tried to develop policies on privileged information, these efforts have been to establish procedures for data protection, not to resolve the issues of which specific information will be released. Section 1166 of the PSRO law, which deals with confidentiality, offers little policy guidance; the law merely sets out in rather broad terms the program's commitment to protect collected data from release.

The statute empowers the Secretary of HEW to develop confidentiality policies sensitive to individual privacy, which means that regulations must be the vehicle for detailing specific requirements. The PSRO in the information area is caught between the positions of full disclosure and nondisclosure, and the law is broad enough to support either position. The fact that presently developing HEW regulations seem to favor selective disclosure does not by any means indicate that the policy would not change with a new Secretary of HEW, an alteration in public opinion, or a successful court challenge. The present PSRO confidentiality policy is fluid and may only be solidified by amending the statute.

This chapter will explore common and statutory law relevant to privacy and confidentiality as it affects peer review operations, whether

131

PSRO or private, and the debate over what information to release or withhold. After identifying basic concepts and trends, we will focus on the law of privacy and confidentiality, from its origins in the physician-patient privilege to its present status in constitutional law. The following sections will discuss the BQA confidentiality guidelines as presently constituted, the Freedom of Information Act, and the Privacy Act, the last two being major pieces of federal legislation that may have a significant impact on PSRO information policy. It should be noted throughout that privacy law is, in many respects, still being developed, so that the protections currently relied upon may be significantly altered by future legal changes.

GENERAL BACKGROUND

The concept of privacy has evolved from a narrowly defined right into a fundamental constitutional guarantee only within the last decade. The growth of technology which has allowed for massive record-keeping systems has created a need to provide protection against invasions into an individual's personal life. While concerns for the protection of privacy are neither new nor unique to our society,[1] the current capacity to collect and store information, as well as the demand for personal information, have dramatically increased. Arthur Miller summarized this trend in his article, "A Nation of Datamaniacs":

Americans today are scrutinized, measured, watched and questioned more than at any time in their history. This increase in data gathering, combined with ever broader applications of information technology, understandably has caused growing anxiety over the erosion of our physical and informational privacy. One major concern is that the computer, with its insatiable appetite for information, its image of infallibility and its inability to forget anything that has been put into it, may become the heart of a surveillance system that will turn society into a transparent world.[2]

Charles Renshaw agreed, and added: "We as a society are confronted with a direct conflict between the need to know, on the one hand, and the desire for privacy on the other. The craving for privacy, it would seem, has become a visceral need in an overcrowded world."[3] Some attempts are being made by most data-gatherers to provide protection for the individual. The most meaningful protections for individual privacy, however, have come from the law—both state and federal legislation—rather than from safeguards developed through private initiative.

Privacy is often defined as one's right to keep information about oneself inaccessible from others. While the definition is accurate, it gives the concept of privacy a theoretical unity lacking in reality. Privacy is not one specific right, but emcompasses a number of considerations and protections that may differ in character. Basically, the right of privacy can be split into two broad classifications: the right of selective disclosure, and the right of physical autonomy. Selective disclosure involves an individual's ability to determine when, how, and to what extent information about the self is communicated to others. The right of physical autonomy is concerned with an individual's ability to determine whether to perform certain acts or undergo certain experiences; it is a right that may protect the physical body or the environment directly around the individual.

In this chapter, the right of selective disclosure is of primary interest, as our concern is with the protection of documented medical information. This does not mean that physical autonomy is not an important right in a medical context. Recognition of this type of privacy was essential in defining a woman's autonomy in the Supreme Court abortion decisions.

While privacy and confidentiality are similar concepts, it should be noted that they are not identical. Privacy, as indicated above, is generally a right of individual protection. Confidentiality, on the other hand, is a right shared by two or more individuals. What confidentiality entails is the protection of any communication made between two or more people (whereas privacy may preclude any type of communication). The communication is protected, not because of the type of information exchanged, but because of the kind of relationship existing between the parties. In most jurisdictions the law recognizes the need for attorneys and clients, priests and penitents, and physicians and patients to develop their relationships in an atmosphere that protects the privacy of information exchanged for professional reasons.

There are few areas in which the issue of privacy and confidentiality is more relevant, or at least more controversial, than in the medical field. While physicians generally recognize that they have a duty, stemming from the Hippocratic Oath, to hold treatment information in confidence, there is no consensus about the extent of that duty. Most physicians would argue that exchange of medical information is vital for adequate treatment, particularly in today's medicine when a single case may be handled by a group of different specialists. Others may argue that, while exchanging information is vital in the treatment setting, storing medical information in data banks to facilitate information exchange destroys the physician-patient confidentiality relationship and puts personal medical information in the hands of a host of people who have little concern for the patient's sensitivity.[4]

The consensus lies somewhere between the extremes of full disclosure and complete nondisclosure of medical information. The current nature of medical practice requires a certain amount of open access to personal medical information. The law has encouraged privacy in dealings between doctor and patient, but has never taken the position that this communication must be protected at all costs, for courts have recognized societal needs that outweigh individual rights.[5]

The medical community alone does not determine what information should be collected, stored or released: much of what occurs in this area reflects the attitudes of society as a whole. The stigma against disclosure of sensitive medical procedures has in many cases been removed with changes in societal attitudes. Certain areas, however, particularly psychiatric treatment, are still considered too sensitive for disclosure; in such cases, legal sanctions are applied against those who release privileged information.*[6]

There is no question that there are a large number of data-gatherers anxious to collect, store and generate medical information in direct challenge to the rights of individual patients. It has been estimated that the federal government alone holds approximately forty million medical records.[7] Insurance companies have large data banks or access to shared data banks which contain personal patient information of a clinical and financial nature on a scale equal to that of the federal government. Insurers need adequate information for business purposes; but whether patients appreciate the fact that insurers have access to their entire medical file, and often share such information with other insurers, is open to question. While the individual may sign a "release of information" form allowing the insurer to examine her/his medical records, many individuals probably do not understand the extent of the release. Even assuming that they do, individuals who need health insurance have little choice in signing such a release.

Unfortunate incidents do occur where data is used to deny an individual insurance coverage or prevent the individual from bringing suit. In a case involving the stealing of medical records, a Denver, Colorado, dis-

---

*In an article in *Trial Magazine,* the justification for privacy in psychiatry is explained: "the very nature of the psychotherapeutic process is based upon free and unrestrained communication between patient and psychiatrist. Any apprehension that statements made might be leaked or publicized would inhibit the whole procedure and make succesful treatment doubtful."

trict attorney stated that "getting medical records is useful for insurance companies and lawyers in heading off lawsuits. In injury cases if an insurance company knows a person has been treated for venereal disease or a psychiatric ailment, the individual may be persuaded not to sue or to accept a lower settlement out of fear the information would come out publicly in court."[8]

Within the medical treatment setting itself the disclosure of patient data is extensive. A patient's hospital record may be handled by a host of health providers, some of whom have little to do with the patient's treatment. In the average hospital the flow of medical information is generally considered to be more important than the strict adherence to patient privacy. The number of individuals involved in treatment make it difficult to prevent broad disclosure of what may be sensitive medical information.

The other major issue in the area of medical privacy is the practitioner's right to protect personally identifiable data. The government collects large amounts of information about physicians for purposes of Titles V, XVIII, and XIX, as do health insurers for payment purposes. With the development of interest in health matters on the part of consumer groups, there has been increasing pressure to disclose the information about physicians' practices for public scrutiny. Physician groups have recently become quite concerned with the issues of privacy, including, in part, their own vulnerability. In the past, a practitioner's behavior was made public through either voluntary release of information or some type of court action. While physicians may release patient information in a variety of ways to fellow physicians, insurers, etc., the release of information about an individual physician's practice outside of litigation was rare. Within hospitals, foundations, and HMOs, various committees have been assembling data on staff physicians' practices, but such information was collected to measure internal institutional behavior; its existence outside the hospital was not widely known.

With the development of peer review programs, information dealing with practitioner behavior patterns is being widely collected. The information is not just assembled, as new data, but is subject to analysis by the review groups, and results in the production of a medical "profile." While the value of a profile is related to the accuracy of the abstracting technique used and may have more significance in some specialties than in others, it represents a unique data-collection effort in which the results can be interpreted to reflect directly on the type of medicine a physician practices.[9]

The practitioner profile, unlike other medical data, allows an objective evaluation of performance and presents information that may be very valuable to both physicians and consumers.[10]

The peer review process, whether under the auspices of the PSRO program, state or federal utilization review, JCAH audit, or other agency, collects, stores, and generates information on all the major actors in the health care system. Whether peer review programs will lead to the release of large amounts of privileged data is largely a matter of speculation, but it is clear that the chances for release are increased.[11]

LEGAL BACKGROUND

The legal doctrine of medical confidentiality developed from the law of evidence, emanating from the physician-patient testimonial privilege. This particular privilege allows a patient who is a witness in court the discretion to withhold personal medical evidence at trial as long as such evidence was developed during the individual's treatment.[12] The justification for the doctor-patient privilege is to encourage freedom of disclosure by patients to physicians during treatment and to protect the patient from embarassment and invasion of privacy. In order for the privilege to apply, the patient must have consulted his own physician (or one he was referred to) for treatment or diagnosis; therefore, the information generated by a court-appointed doctor or one selected by an insurance company does not fall within this privilege.

In recent years, the testimonial privilege has fallen out of favor and has been substantially eroded by developments in other evidentiary areas. From a jurist's standpoint, the doctor-patient privilege has been far from satisfactory in eliciting complete and accurate trial testimony. Use of the privilege results in the suppression of the best source of proof, the examining and treating physician who could most accurately testify on the patient's physical or mental condition. Such criticism has resulted in a significant modification of the doctor-patient privilege; for example, the judge may compel disclosure when it is felt necessary for proper judicial administration.[13] The trend in most jurisdictions is toward complete abandonment of the privilege.[14]

Litigation Based Upon the Breach of Physician-Patient Relationship

It is from the doctor-patient testimonial privilege that a cause of action for unauthorized disclosure arose in the common law. In jurisdictions with a statute including the testimonial privilege, there has been an almost uniform recognition of suits based on confidentiality breaches. For example, in *Clark v. Geraci*,[15] an action against a physician for disclosing information obtained in a professional capacity, a New York court said that, "While no principle of common law is violated by such disclosure, it is plainly reprehensible as indicated by the statutory law regulating physicians' conduct, accepted usage . . . information possessed by a doctor of the illness of his patient has long been thought of as protected professional confidence upon which the patient may rely."[16]

In jurisdictions which have not enacted a testimonial privilege statute, the development of suits based on confidentiality breaches have been fairly well split. The Supreme Court of New Jersey, a jurisdiction not recognizing the testimonial privilege, in the case of *Hague v. Williams*[17] made a distinction between testimonial and non-testimonial disclosures. The New Jersey court reasoned that the relationship between doctor and patient created a duty for the physician not to disclose to persons outside the judiciary information obtained in confidence.

The testimonial privilege is not the sole basis for actions on breaches of physician confidentiality; other statutory and public policy grounds come into play in this development. In the case of *Simonsen v. Swenson* (1920)[18] the Nebraska court found that the physician's duty to hold information in confidence was derived from a general legal duty of secrecy: "A wrongful breach of such confidence (physician-patient) and a betrayal of such trust would give rise to a civil action for the damages naturally flowing from such wrong."[19]

The Supreme Court of Alabama, in its encompassing opinion dealing with the physician-patient privilege in *Horne v. Patton*,[20] enunciated a strong public policy development that, coupled with a statutory basis (either testimonial privilege or licensure laws), resulted in a legally sanctioned cloak of confidentiality over the doctor-patient relationship. The court's public policy argument stems from the Hippocratic Oath and Principle 9 of the AMA Code of Ethics, both of which entrust the physician with a duty of confidentiality unless the public welfare necessitates otherwise. In the words of the Supreme Court of Alabama, "when the wording of the state licensing statute is considered alongside the accepted precepts of the medical profession itself, it would seem to establish clearly that public policy in Alabama requires that information obtained by a physician in the course of a doctor-patient relationship be maintained unless the patient demands otherwise.[21]

Some courts have held that the physician-patient relationship is a contractual one from which springs an implied condition that information will be kept confidential. It was stated in a discussion of the physician-patient contract in *Hammonds v. Aetna Casualty and Surety Company* that "an implied condition of the physician-patient contract, this court is of the opinion that the doctor warrants that any confidential information gained through the relationship will not be released without the patient's permission . . . every patient has a right to rely on this warranty of silence . . . when a doctor breaches his duty of secrecy, he is in violation of part of his obligations under the contract."[22] The Supreme Court of Alabama in *Horne v. Patton* reinforced the Hammonds decision, upholding what it referred to as the reasonable expectations on the part of the patient to keep confidential all information transferred by the individual as a contractual right.[23]

The Law of Privacy

While the right of privacy as a separate cause of action in the common law was first posited in the 1880's, broader development of the right has occurred only within the last thirty years. Privacy has often been recognized in tort law as protecting a number of specific interests, such as freedom from mental distress, protection of reputation, and the proprietary interest in one's name or likeness. The limited approach does not advance the privacy concept as a protected interest in and of itself, for dividing "privacy" into a series of litigable categories reflects consequences of invasion to one's personality but does not establish a separate right. A patient damaged by a breach of privacy had to proceed against his physician on a theory that required demonstration of a violation of a narrowly defined interest such as freedom from mental distress, protection of reputation, etc.

Eventually, the concept of privacy has come to be recognized by most American jurisdictions as an independent cause of action not based on some specifically protected interest. Litigation protecting personality has developed the privacy doctrine primarily in the context of the rights of citizens to prevent disclosure of information by the media; it rests on a flexible basis that tests the extent and reasonableness of the intrusion. In jurisdictions that have recognized the individual right of privacy as an independent cause of action, patient plaintiffs have sued physicians who have released personally identifiable medical information without the patient's consent. As a result of these suits, there have been instances where the court held a patient's privacy to have been violated even though the medical information taken was not published.[24]

The Supreme Court and Privacy

The U.S. Supreme Court has in recent years developed a constitutionally sanctioned right of privacy that has important implications for the physician-patient relationship and for medical practice in general. Clearly, in the words of the Constitution there is no doctrine that responds to the intense pressures placed upon the individual's freedom in modern society. While the right of privacy was extrapolated from the law, we sometimes feel that it was a right created out of necessity rather than on a clear legal foundation. The dual concept of privacy (selective disclosure and personal autonomy), while not mentioned by the Court as such, is helpful to remember in any analysis of the constitutional doctrine of privacy, for the right seems to develop around one or both of these concepts.

The early Supreme Court decisions dealing with privacy focused on protecting the physical environment, and gradually moved toward a general right with recognizing associational, political, and bodily privacy. A landmark decision in the development of a constitutionally recognized right of privacy was handed down in 1965 in *Griswold v. Connecticut*.[25] In this case, the Court struck down a state criminal statute that prohibited the use of contraceptives as violating individual autonomy and the right of selective disclosure. Justice Douglas identified a constitutional right of privacy based upon rights emanating from the 1st, 4th, and 9th amendments (penumbral rights). Thus the privacy right, while not expressed, was deemed to be rooted in the spirit of the Bill of Rights. The Griswold case recognized privacy as a constitutional right in a marital context, but before long the scope of this right was expanded.[26] In the Court's words, "It is true that in Griswold the right of privacy in question inhered in the marital relationship. Yet the marital couple is not an independent entity with a mind and heart of its own, but an association of two individuals each with separate intellectual and emotional makeup. If the right of privacy means anything, it is the right of the individual, married or single, to be free from unwarranted government intrusion."[27]

The Supreme Court's approach to the constitutional right of privacy was altered in its 1973 abortion decisions. In *Roe v. Wade*,[28] the Court struck down a Texas criminal statute that prevented abortion and arrived at a concept of privacy much broader than that expressed in the Griswold case. The Roe decision extended the protection of privacy to any area where the protection is required to safeguard the intimacy of the activity involved. What occurred was a transformation of the privacy theory based upon an amalgamation of principles in the Bill of Rights to a singularly independent concept of personal liberty which places a limit on the ability of the state to restrict individual autonomy in certain instances. For even with the abortion cases, the Court has not supplied an adequate definition of the overall privacy right, but merely delineated a catalog approach of those activities that are to be protected. The Court does not recognize that all activities should receive the blanket protection of privacy: in *Paris Adult Theatre I v. Slaton,*[29] a Georgia statute prohibiting the distribution of obscene films was upheld as constitutional and not infringing on an individual's privacy right.

Justice Douglas's concurrence in the Roe abortion case placed heavy emphasis on the physician-patient relationship as being crucial to the right of privacy; this recognition gives credence to independent causes of action for breach of physician-patient confidentialities. Douglas wrote, "The right of privacy—the right to care for one's health and person and to seek out a physician of one's own choice—is protected by the XIV Amendment."[30] The abortion decisions protect the right of privacy of the physician as well as the mother, giving the former the ability to administer medical treatment according to professional judgment. The constitutional recognition of the physician-patient relationship as a private one relates both to selective disclosure and personal autonomy of the individual concerning his health status. The Court's determination that the medical treatment situation was (at least in some instances) protected by a constitutional guarantee of privacy has significant implications for constructing an argument that medical peer review may be unconstitutional. (See Chapter 4.)

While the Supreme Court has taken significant steps in establishing the privacy right, that right is afforded only when a tangible or measurable injury is present. The Court has not yet recognized the creation of massive data banks which contain highly personal information as constituting in and of themselves a violation of personal privacy. In the case of *Laird v. Tatum,*[31] the Court rejected the notion that an army data bank dealing with the political activities of private citizens violated a right to privacy, because no tangible injury was present. Neither the collection of personal information nor the existence of the record-keeping system was found by the court to constitute injury. A legal journal noted that, "The Court in Tatum refused to grant relief from the alleged injuries to the spirit and the psyche; it refused to admit that maintenance of data banks could cause anything more than a subjective chill of plaintiff's constitutional rights."[32] Justice Douglas in a dissent in the Tatum case argued that the very existence of a massive data-gathering system was a threat to privacy.[33]

In *California Bankers Association v. Schultz*,[34] the Court again ruled that the mere existence of a data bank, in this case held by the banking industry, did not in and of itself cause injury to the individual. It is evident from the two cases cited above that the Court does not yet recognize privacy as a free-standing right based on the existence of potential damage caused by a breach of one's privacy.*

Freedom of Information Act and Privacy Act

As far as federal legislation is concerned, two bills that affect the protection of medical information are the Freedom of Information Act (FOIA)[35] and the Privacy Act of 1974.[36] The relationship between these two bills and the PSRO organization will be discussed further on in this chapter.**

The federal FOIA was passed in 1970 to allow citizen access to records kept by federal agencies. The act replaced §3 of the Administrative Procedures Act, which had made it discretionary with federal agencies as to whether or not they would release information. The Freedom of Information Act placed the burden upon the agencies to demonstrate why identifiable records should not be released. A recent amendment to the act has made it more workable for information seekers by broadening the term "identifiable" and setting a time limit within which the agency must comply. The act is not, however, a blanket pass to agency information, for a number of exemptions have been included in the statute to protect certain classes of sensitive information.[37]

The Privacy Act of 1974 represents the first large-scale legislative attempt to protect the personal privacy rights of individual citizens from abuse by government agencies. The Privacy Act places safeguards on the misuse of information held by federal agencies and federal contractors engaged in carrying out agency functions. Under the Privacy Act four main objectives can be identified: (1) to insure fairness to individuals when agencies are making decisions based on personal data, (2) to limit access to identifiable agency records, (3) to insure accuracy of personal data, and (4) to establish a mechanism for public accountability for record holders.

One commentator noted that, "In general, the Act adopts the philosophy that identifiable information shall not be disclosed without the informed consent of the individual to whom the record pertains."[38] Agen-

---

*See *Whalen v. Roe*, U. S. Law Week No. 75–839 (1977).

**The government in the Sunshine Act passed in 1976 will not be discussed in this chapter. The Sunshine Act requires federal agencies to have meetings open to the public unless the topic falls within one of the statute's ten exemptions. (P.L. 94–409).

cies are required by the Privacy Act to publish in the *Federal Register* annual listings of their existing record-keeping systems, and notices must also be published concerning proposals for new uses of data and of new record-keeping systems. The Privacy Act lists a number of exceptions which permit a federal agency to release information without the identifiable party's consent: for example, under the federal Freedom of Information Act, by court order, for routine agency use, etc. The Privacy Act discourages the use of joint or shared data bases between agencies and encourages where possible the obtaining of personal data directly from the individual rather than from another agency.[39] An agency is limited to the collection of data that it feels is necessary to perform a specific task.

Under the Privacy Act an individual has the right to find out whether a given agency is collecting information on him, to gain access to his record, and to obtain a copy of the record.[40] In the case of medical records, an agency may establish special access procedures so that an individual's physician representative can be given a copy of the medical record.[41] In the event that an individual challenges the information contained in an agency file as being inaccurate or incomplete, the information can be reviewed by the agency to determine whether or not the record is correct.[42] An individual who feels that an agency has improperly denied him access to a record may bring a legal action under the Privacy Act against the agency seeking injunctive relief, damages, or an amendment of the record.[43]

While the Privacy Act is a significant first step toward protecting individual privacy, the Act fails to include data systems held by private organizations, as well as information held by local and state governments. One problem, identified by Professor Boyer in his *Buffalo Law Review* article on the Privacy Act is: "the Act does not attempt to deal with the risk that organizations with economic leverage or other forms of power over the individual data subject will use this advantage to compel the individual to obtain copies of his records and submit them with applications for benefits. Since medical records are often relevant to employment or credit granting decisions, and since government agencies ranging from military to the Medicare program collect large quantities of medical information, this risk may not be insubstantial."[44]

State Law

In examining the questions of privacy and confidentiality of peer review records, it is important to note that PSROs fall under the control of federal regulation, and therefore that state policies concerning privileged data are probably not applicable. State law is preempted by federal law when there is conflict or the possibility of conflict between them, but not otherwise. In other review programs, including those run by a state Medicaid agency or a private Foundation for Medical Care, state law will apply to issues of data access.

While the policies adopted by the states on access to medical records lack consistency, there are certain general situations where release of patient records routinely occurs, especially in the acute-care facility. When a patient enters a hospital he often signs a form that allows the institution to release medical information to whomever it feels has a legitimate need for such information. Medical records can be released to payment agencies (fiscal intermediary or welfare departments) for hospital procurement purposes, or to a hospital cost-monitoring agency.[45] Within the institution itself there is thought to be an implied consent that individuals involved in a patient's care have a right to examine the individual's record; these individuals include anyone from the ward secretary to the attending physician. A hospital medical review committee has an implied consent to examine and review a patient's medical record.[46] Information in medical records is routinely released to fulfill public reporting statutes (vital statistics, dangerous diseases, etc.). In a lawsuit where a party's physical condition is at issue, the medical record can be subpoenaed for use in court. Finally, a physician may release medical information about a patient when he feels it is in the patient's best interests. For example, the physician has the right to discuss the patient's condition with members of the patient's family without receiving prior consent.

The question of access to or release of utilization review and audit committee minutes, records, and profiles presents a different issue: a distinction must be made from the policies developed concerning release of medical records. The records generated by peer review committees, while containing medical information, are not "medical records" from a legal standpoint. Peer review committee records are not made to describe a patient's treatment but to evaluate that treatment.

A significant number of American jurisdictions have passed special legislation to protect medical review committee records.[47] Such state laws provide peer review committees with varying protections, ranging from an absolute denial of discovery and subpoena of records and documentation to a classification of committee records as "privileged"[48] but with no specification as to what such designations mean. An example of fairly broad protective legislation for medical peer review committees is that which has been adopted by the state of Minnesota. The Minnesota statute reads, "All data and information acquired by a review organization, in the exercise of its duties and functions, shall be held in confidence, shall not be disclosed to anyone except to the extent necessary to carry out one or more of the purposes of the review organization and shall not be subject to subpoena or discovery."[49]

While the amount of litigation dealing with the discovery of medical committee records has not been extensive, a number of cases have been litigated on this point based upon either specific state statutes or public policy principles. Perhaps the most widely quoted case resting upon a nonstatutory basis is *Breddice v. Doctor's Hospital*,[50] in which a federal court ruled against disclosure of hospital committee minutes and reports as being in contradiction with the public interest. The court in the Breddice case stated that "confidentiality is essential to effective functioning of these staff meetings, and these staff meetings are essential to the continued improvement in the care and treatment of patients . . . to subject these discussions and deliberations to the discovery process, without a showing of exceptional necessity, would result in terminating such deliberations."[51] In the Arizona case of *Jolly v. Superior Court of Pinal County*,[52] the public policy rationale for classifying medical committee records as privileged was similarly expressed. The Arizona court reasoned that, "The privilege of protecting medical committee records is justified by the overwhelming public interest . . . so that the flow of ideas and advice may continue unimpeded and the quality of medical care and treatment may be enhanced."[53]

In *Matchett v. Superior Court for the County of Yuba*,[54] a California Court of Appeals upheld a state statute that barred discovery of hospital committee records of those committees responsible for evaluating and improving the institution's quality of care.[55] While the California court supported the public interest rationale in barring discovery, it recognized a difficulty in holding such a position: "this confidentiality exacts a social cost, because it impairs a malpractice plaintiff's access to evidence. In a damage suit for inhospital malpractice against doctor or hospital or both, unavailability of recorded evidence of incompetence might seriously jeopardize or even prevent the plaintiff's recovery. Section 1157 of the California Evidence Code represents a legislative choice between competing public concerns. It embraces the goal of medical staff candor at the cost of impairing plaintiff's access to evidence."[56]

In the New Jersey case of *Young v. King*,[57] the court ruled that only the minutes and reports of the hospital utilization review committee were exempt from discovery proceedings, because only that committee was specifically mentioned in the New Jersey statute.[58] The Young case is interesting because the court, in strictly adhering to a statute, failed to protect other hospital committee records (such as those of tissue and audit committees) which may, in fact, be considerably more sensitive than U.R. committee documentation. While special state statutes may act in a varying degree to protect medical peer review committee records from discovery or subpoena, the nature of those records may affect the question of accessibility.

State "Freedom of Information" Acts

Many American jurisdictions have some type of Freedom of Information statute, often called a "right to know" law, that allows for access to records held by state agencies. It must be noted that only medical records collected by the state are subject to state Freedom of Information laws; therefore, the review committees established under a state Medicaid program may be subject to such a law, but PSRO review committees are not. State Freedom of Information laws require state agencies to allow members of the public the right to examine and copy records held by state government.[59]

Like their federal counterpart,[60] state Freedom of Information laws contain a number of exempt categories. Medical records are specified as an exempt category in many state Freedom of Information statutes, but whether that category is broad enough to include review committee records is a matter of judicial discretion. It can be argued, based on the statutory language used in many state Freedom of Information acts, that the term "medical record" should not be limited to a statutorily defined hospital or physician office record, but should include all types of sensitive medical information.

For example, the New York State law exempts the "disclosure of items involving the medical or personal records of a client or patient in a hospital or medical facility."[61] This would seem broad enough to include peer review committee records.[62] While access to committee records may be possible under state Freedom of Information statutes, the limitation of application (state-collected records only) and the exemptions placed upon release of medical records by these state statutes may, in fact, render them of little value in obtaining peer review documents.

State Consumer Protection Laws

It may be possible to obtain peer review committee records by use of state consumer protection laws.[63] In examining state consumer protection laws, one may note that they are, ordinarily, modeled directly after provisions of the Federal Trade Commission Act. The section of state consumer protection laws that is of special interest in the peer review context is the provision dealing with unfair and deceptive practices.[64]

Section 349 (a) of the General Business Law of New York State reads, "Deceptive acts or practices in the conduct of any business, trade or commerce or in the furnishing of any service in this state are hereby declared unlawful."[65] This statute represents a typical example of a consumer protection law. In order to establish an argument for release of medical peer review committee records, two key elements must be proved beyond the applicability of the statute: first, the review body must be considered to be engaged in a trade or business, and, second, there must be an injury caused by failure to release information recognized by the statute.

While one may argue that failure to release peer review committee records constitutes an unfair and deceptive practice, the question must first be answered whether review committees in hospitals or foundations could be considered to fall under these regulations. Massachusetts law (GL Chapter 93A, Section 1) defines trade and commerce as "the distribution of any services . . . and any other thing of value . . . and shall include any trade . . . indirectly affecting the people of this Commonwealth."[66] In a consumer report prepared by the Harvard Center for Community Health,[67] it was argued that the PSROs were an organization engaged in trade or commerce: "Promulgation of quality assurance controls, with the concomitant right to withhold payment from practitioners and providers failing to meet PSRO guidelines, represents a direct and substantial economic impact on and intervention in the trade of its membership."[68]

Such an argument could be drawn, by analogy, to state medical review programs. It is not necessary to do so, however, since most of the other review groups are part of a corporate entity (such as a hospital, foundation) which is clearly engaged in a trade or business. The review committee, while not directly dealing with the consumer, is part of an organization affected by consumer protection legislation.[69]

The question of classifying the withholding of medical review committee information as a type of injury covered under state Consumer Protection Laws raises a fundamental question of the effect of peer review committee data. The consumer position is that medical peer review data is required in order for individuals to make intelligent choices about their own health care, and that the failure to obtain such data causes injury to the patient/consumer. Whether a court would agree that peer review committee data is needed by consumers to make health care choices depends upon the types and extent of information generated by committees. It would presently take a rather liberal court to agree that the need of the consumer to obtain peer review data is more important than the maintenance of the confidentiality of medical peer review.[70]

Consumer protection laws have created grounds for suit for unfair and deceptive practices not available under the common law, but one can question whether the withholding of information is unfair or deceptive. Consumer statutes are oriented toward protecting the individual in a business or commercial context. The California Consumer Legal Remedies Act lists eighteen unfair and deceptive practices as being unlawful, and none of the eighteen would cover failure to disclose medical information.[71] The California consumer law's unfair and deceptive practices section, as in other state laws is oriented toward violations that require a positive act of misrepresentation, which may be difficult to discern from a hospital's, HMO's, or foundation's unwillingness to release peer review committee data.

In Massachusetts, however, the state Supreme Court, in the case of *Commonwealth v. DeCotis,*[72] ruled in interpreting the Massachusetts Consumer Protection Law that "this act is one of several legislative attempts in recent years to regulate business activities with a view to providing proper disclosure of information."[73] Therefore, in the eyes of the Massachusetts courts, withholding peer review information would probably constitute an unfair or deceptive practice. In interpreting the DeCotis case it seems that monetary damages need be only nominal for the injury to form the basis of injunctive relief.[74]

The question of the effect of state consumer protection laws on release of medical peer review committee data will ultimately be answered in state courts. The applicability of such statutes may be quite limited as a result of state laws limiting discovery of such records. Other limiting factors are the small number of medical review programs affected by consumer statutes and the vagueness of the types of injury allegedly caused by failure to release medical committee information.

PSRO CONFIDENTIALITY POLICY

The PSRO is caught in a debate between two major forces in the confidentiality area: one force seeks the release of all information, regardless of whether or not it is personally identifiable; the other holds that no PSRO data should be disclosed, for once released, the organization has no control over how the information is used. It is between these two extremes that the Bureau of Quality Assurance (BQA) is attempting to develop policies for access and disclosure. As indicated earlier, PSRO confidentiality policy is largely left to the discretion of the Secretary of

HEW, for the law is too general to offer guidance in specific areas.[75] This section discusses policy drawn from transmittal Letter No. 16 and various draft guidelines, all used as a basis for regulations in this area.

It is important to note that the regulatory law governing confidentiality is susceptible to change because the law's statutory base will support both extremes of the access-and-disclosure question. Indeed, one could make a reasonable public policy argument to release all physician profiles which would probably be as persuasive to a court as the present policy of protecting identifiable physician data.[76] The present confidentiality policy is also subject to change because loopholes in the system will emerge. For example, institutional data was not originally thought to be protected, but its release was to be left to PSRO discretion. Under the interim confidentiality regulations (Dec. 3, 1976, 41 F.R. 234), only aggregate UHDDS data is to be released which cannot be traced to an individual; this position represents a modification of Transmittal 41 policy, which prohibited the release of any hospital data outside the PSRO system.[77]

The PSRO confidentiality policy as outlined at this time is only the first of several policies that BQA will develop for handling sensitive data. The Bureau of Quality Assurance, while attempting to balance the competing interests of open disclosure and no disclosure, is bound to come into conflict with one or both of the parties involved in this dispute. BQA regulatory policy will probably lead to both litigation and a series of amended regulations that may result in significant changes in some areas of disclosure policy.[78]

When considering the PSRO confidentiality question, our initial concern is to identify "privileged information" in the context of the PSRO program. BQA policy is that any information held by a PSRO that is personally identifiable to a patient or physician is privileged. Information used in the development of a medical care evaluation study (MCE) that is not routinely collected for review purposes, as well as records of PSRO committee determinations are also privileged. As far as the institution is concerned, identifiable information will not be protected. Public and legal pressure is too great to prevent a policy of nondisclosure. HSA pressure lead to development of BQA policy leading to release of aggregate hospital data.* Special procedures are to be set up to allow an institution to comment about identifiable information which has been requested.[79]

---

*Specifications for regulations on confidentiality issued March 1, 1977 indicate that hospital data other than contained in MCEs will be subject to disclosure. Hospitals will have the opportunity to supply accompanying comment.

Individual patients, physicians, or institutions on whom the PSRO is collecting, storing, and generating information will have the right of access to their own records for the purpose of determining their accuracy. The PSRO is required to develop special access procedures. In the case of patient access, the physician of record is to be notified 15 days prior to the access. The physician of record does not have the ability to prevent any of his patients from accessing their own records, but does have the right to be present at the time the patient examines the record to make appropriate clarifications. The patient who examines his record will be required to sign a form testifying to the fact he has received a copy of his PSRO profile. The PSRO should inform the patient about the nature of the PSRO record, i.e., that it is less complete than the hospital medical record. The PSRO must present profiles to any requesting party in a version that has been translated from code into readable text, because the coded document on its face would be of little value to most individuals. Elderly patients or others unable for whatever reason to examine their records may appoint a representative to do so.

In the case of a minor who wishes to see his record, BQA policy allows for access, but recommends that in such a case the attending physician or a physician appointed by the PSRO be present to explain the record to the minor. The parents or guardian of a minor may have access to information in a minor's record by designating a physician to review the record on the PSRO premises. HEW guidelines state: The PSRO should discuss the request for access with the physician of record or, should he be unavailable, with the PSRO Medical Director or other physician officer of the PSRO and determine if disclosure of the information in the PSRO file would constitute an invasion of the privacy of the individual under 18."[80]

There are several additional instances in which privileged PSRO records will be disclosed. In both the appeals and sanction proceedings, any of the involved parties will have the right to examine privileged PSRO profiles and committee records relevant to the case at hand. If a physician is actually sanctioned, that fact becomes a matter of public record, but how extensive this disclosure will be has not yet been determined.[81] Most disclosures of privileged PSRO information will occur to fulfill state and federal reporting requirements for monitoring, review, and evaluation purposes. It should be noted that while privileged PSRO information will be disclosed in certain instances, privileged material generally cannot be physically removed from the PSRO premises. "Privileged information or data may not be physically removed and/or transmitted outside of the PSRO review system except for the purposes of appeals or sanctions."[82]

Privileged information held by the PSRO may be of interest to trial attorneys in certain types of litigation. For instance, in a medical malpractice case a PSRO's physician profile may help demonstrate a pattern of practitioner incompetence.[83] The general rule developed by HEW exempts privileged PSRO information from subpoena, thus preventing the use of such information in discovery proceedings or at trial. Similarly, an individual working in the PSRO cannot be called upon to testify about privileged material of which he has knowledge. The only exception to the ban against subpoena would be in cases dealing with review determination that have been pursued in a federal court; the PSRO record would be essential to such a case and is not protected from such subpoena by the guidelines.

RESPONSIBILITIES OF THE PSRO CONCERNING PRIVILEGED DATA

Each PSRO has a duty to inform the public at least once a year in the local press about the PSRO's information-gathering function: namely, that it is collecting, storing, and generating medical information, and that it has developed procedures for access and protection of information. A more specific type of notice must be provided to those individuals and institutions about whom the PSRO has collected information. This notice should detail: (1) the individual in the PSRO who will be responsible for ensuring confidentiality, (2) the individual who will have access to privileged PSRO data, and, (3) specific access procedures adopted by the PSRO.

The PSRO is required to designate one individual within its organization as the confidentiality coordinator who will be in charge of maintaining confidentiality and adequate security over PSRO data. The confidentiality coordinator will be responsible for developing, implementing, and monitoring a plan to insure that confidentiality measures are enforced; will report violations of security to HEW; will maintain records of disclosure and authorized access; and will coordinate employee confidentiality training programs. Each unit of the PSRO is required to develop its own confidentiality statement, which is to be reviewed by the confidentiality coordinator to insure that it complies with the organization's overall policy.

The PSRO's individual officers and employees will be required to undergo a training program dealing with PSRO confidentiality procedures prior to their being able to access privileged information. Employees and officers will also be required to sign a statement confirming their awareness of the sensitive nature of PSRO data and of the penalty for unauthorized disclosure.

The PSRO may wish to make a special agreement with delegated hospitals to the effect that the latter will abide by the PSRO confidentiality policy where individuals performing review are hospital employees. Subcontractors of the PSRO involved in data processing must develop specific procedures that will guarantee confidentiality of the information they handle.[84]

While a PSRO employee or officer may have clearance to examine privileged data, this access must be necessary to perform a specific task. In other words, privileged data must be accessed with a clear "need to know" on the part of the PSRO individual examining the data. HEW guidelines state that, "Need to know disclosures give a person 'just enough' information and no more to carry out his or her assigned functions. These assigned functions should be compatible and associated with the limited purposes for which the information is collected."[85] Each time PSRO privileged data is accessed, the incident of access must be recorded on some type of log.

Identification of patients, physicians, and hospitals or other health institutions on PSRO records and forms will be codified, with Social Security numbers used as identifiers by most PSROs, although separate codes may be developed. The PSRO's indexing files' cross referencing identifier codes should receive the highest degree of protection. PSRO documents, tapes, printouts, or punch cards considered to be privileged must be marked as such and stored in a secure, fire-proof area. When the privileged information is no longer of value for monitoring, evaluation, review, or appeals purposes, it is to be purged; computer files, however, may be maintained indefinitely.

FEDERAL FREEDOM OF INFORMATION ACT

The PSRO presently falls under the Federal Freedom of Information Act only to a limited extent.[86] Say HEW guidelines, "Reports generated by the PSRO containing information required by Federal agencies in their monitoring and program review capacity are considered to come under the Freedom of Information Act and once received by HEW are subject to its disclosure provisions."[87] Only information routinely reported to HEW by a PSRO would fall within the federal disclosure requirements. Release of personally identifiable records would generally not be required by HEW; if such information were needed, it would be subject only to onsite review. There may, however, be instances when sensitive matter will have to be transmitted to HEW, such as sanction situations, and in these cases the Freedom of Information Act may conceivably be used as a vehicle to access such reports.[88]

The Freedom of Information Act has been viewed both as a threat to the PSRO and as a realistic avenue for obtaining access to PSRO records. Whether or not the Freedom of Information Act can be extended to PSROs is a matter that must be judicially determined. The present BQA confidentiality policy may be circumvented by use of this legislation, thus opening access to privileged PSRO data.

To assess the feasibility of applying the FOIA to PSROs, a fundamental legal determination on the status of the PSRO must be made. If one holds that the PSRO is a private, nonprofit state corporation, which is the current federal policy, then the Freedom of Information Act will not apply.[89] However, this discussion assumes for the sake of argument that the PSRO may be, for purposes of the Act, a federal entity. Such interpretation of the PSRO's legal status is reinforced by recent amendments to the Freedom of Information Act (PL. 93-502) which have significantly expanded the definition of "agency."[90]

If the Freedom of Information Act applies to PSROs, we must consider two exemption provisions in this law: (B)(6), which exempts medical files held by federal agencies from disclosures, and (B)(3), which recognizes statutory exemptions. If either of these two exemptions apply, privileged PSRO data may be inaccessible despite the Freedom of Information Act's applicability.

The sensitive information held by the PSRO does not fall within any one statutory category. Some of the PSRO's privileged data may clearly be considered to fall within the classification of "medical file," a category specifically exempted in §(B)(6) of the Act. Certainly, the patient profile could be considered a "medical file," but whether or not other PSRO privileged information would fall into that exemption classification is open to question. In interpreting the medical files-personnel records exemption section in (B)(6), courts have been concerned with the extent of personal invasion. A type of balancing approach has been taken in the interpretation of the (B)(6) records exemption: "The court must first measure the loss of individual privacy that would result from disclosure.

Against that factor must be measured the suitability of the complainant seeking disclosure. The need and status of the discoverant, in addition to the purposes underlying the request, are relevant to establishing suitability."[91] It is thus ultimately left to the federal court to determine whether disclosure of medical files constitutes an unwarranted invasion of personal privacy, and also to settle disputes about whether the exemption was properly invoked.[92] While the word "person" as used in the

Administrative Procedures Act, and hence in this section of the FOIA, does include a corporation, it would seem that exemption (B)(6) of 5 U.S.C. refers specifically to an individual personage.

The second Freedom of Information Act exemption we must consider is that which excludes matter "specifically exempted from disclosure by statute"§(B)(3). This particular exemption may be effective in preventing release of privileged PSRO data, because §1166 of the PSRO law provides statutory authority to the Secretary of HEW to withhold information from disclosure "in such cases and under such circumstances as the Secretary shall by regulations provide to assure adequate protection of the rights and interests of patients, health care practitioners or providers of health care."[93]

The application of the statutory exemption in §(B)(3) of the Freedom of Information Act is not clearcut. On its face, §(B)(3) seems to act as a blanket exemption, but in fact the federal courts have interpreted the section in varying fashion. Some courts have held that FOIA exemptions should be construed quite narrowly in view of the statute's purpose to make government-held information readily accessible.[94] In the case of *Stretch v. Weinberger,* [95] the U.S. Court of Appeals for the 3rd Circuit held that certain reports concerning performance of nursing and old age programs prepared for the Medicare program were not subject to protection via the FOIA exemption provision. The court in the Stretch case reasoned that if the information were to fall under (B)(3), it must be specifically exempted from disclosure by statute.

Specific exemption requires that a statute either identifies some class or category of items that Congress considers appropriate for exemption; or, at least, sets out legislatively prescribed standards for guidelines that the Secretary must follow in determining what matters shall be exempted from disclosure. Not all federal courts have reached the same conclusion as the Stretch court, but the Stretch case and decisions similar to it raise the possibility that (B)(3) may not protect PSRO information.

If the Freedom of Information Act applies, therefore, there is a question whether §1166(a) of the PSRO law is a specific enough basis upon which the Secretary can issue regulations to protect sensitive PSRO data. It can be argued that §1166(a) is overly vague in defining the Secretary's power, for it does not specify which data will be held in confidence, or how determinations of confidentiality will be made. A federal court could very well conclude that the language of §1166(a) is too broad to sustain exemption (B)(3) of the Freedom of Information Act.

It is also possible to argue that releasing certain types of privileged information, such as practitioner profiles or committee records, is necessary to ensure that the PSRO statute is fulfilled, and therefore that information dealing with providers and practitioners must be exempted by the Secretary. On the other hand, a court may feel that a certain flexibility is required by §1166(a) in view of the fact that when the PSRO law was passed, it was not clear what types of records PSROs would be generating.

Finally, it is important to note that the FOIA exemptions are in most instances optional, and it is up to agency discretion whether they will be employed.[96] Whether to release privileged PSRO data (if the (B)(3) and/or (B)(6) exemptions apply) may rest with the Secretary of HEW. The Secretary may decide to release certain privileged information due to public pressure or a belief that release is most consistent with the purposes of a given program.

PRIVACY ACT

The current position of the Bureau of Quality Assurance is that the Privacy Act of 1974 does not apply to the PSRO. However, BQA policy states, "At this time the PSRO program is not subject to the Privacy Act of 1974 . . . the PSRO Confidentiality policy and guidelines have been designed to parallel those of the Privacy Act to the maximum extent possible.[97] The BQA policy statement acknowledges the PSRO fact that compliance with Confidentiality Policy does not constitute compliance with the Privacy Act. If the latter is to apply, additional policy requirements may have to be developed. The BQA statement concerning the Privacy Act is interesting because it seems to assume that the Act will apply in the future.

Section 552A(m) of the Privacy Act applies the Act to federal contractors who are carrying out an agency function. It would seem reasonable to argue that a PSRO, in carrying out its mandate to review the necessity and quality of medical care provided under titles XVIII, XIX, and V of the Social Security Act, could be classified as carrying out an HEW function. The PSRO program, as a federal contractor, can be viewed as an organization designed to aid in the management of SSA funds. On the other hand, if one views the Privacy Act contract provision strictly, it could be argued that the Act applies only to tasks specifically mandated of federal agencies; and as medical review is required of PSROs but not HEW, the contractor provision does not apply. OMB guidelines attempt to limit application of the contractor provision "to those systems directly related to the performance of federal agency functions."[98]

It may, however, be difficult to limit the application of the Privacy Act to PSROs under §552A(m) in view of HEW's position that Medicare intermediaries and carriers are Department agents in performing Medicare functions: "The Department has determined that intermediaries and carriers are agents of the Department (as well as contractors) in carrying out Medicare functions imposed by law on the Secretary and by reason of this agency status are subject to all of the provisions of the Privacy Act."[99]

If the Privacy Act is extended to the PSRO program, the initial effect upon PSRO operations would not be as significant as the application of the Freedom of Information Act. The Privacy Act allows individuals to obtain copies of their records. Under the Privacy Act, alternative access procedures will be established for medical records: copies of medical records may be released to some designated party. Under present PSRO policy, record access can occur, but records can be copied and removed from the PSRO. If the Privacy Act is to apply to the PSROs, patients, physicians, and institutions would have to be given copies of their records. Once copies of PSRO records are made available to the identifiable party, it would be impossible for the PSRO to effectively control how the information was used outside of the PSRO premises.

Under HEW policy for the Privacy Act,[100] an individual has the ability to grant consent to third parties so that they can obtain disclosure of an individual's personal record. The policy states, "An individual may grant consent to the disclosure to third parties of records pertaining to him . . . consent to the disclosure of medical information will be honored only if it is executed not more than 45 days prior to the third party's request for access to the record."[101] Clearly, under the PSRO system as it presently stands, an individual does not have the authority to allow third parties to examine his record, with the exception of an attending or other physician representative.

If the PSRO is governed by the Privacy Act, that statute's exemption section, which allows for the disclosure of individual records in a limited number of cases without prior consent, may be germane. Three of the exemption categories in the Privacy Act have a potential effect upon PSROs: exemptions for disclosure under the Freedom of Information Act, court subpoena of information, and routine use of data in agency operations.[102] Assuming that all of these exemptions listed apply to the PSRO if it falls under the Privacy Act, the most difficult one to deal with would be the "routine use" exemption. The Privacy Act defines "routine use" as use of a record for purposes compatible with the reasons for which the record was collected. It is difficult to determine on the basis of this definition what criteria a court would use in deciphering what a "compatible" record use would be. One could, for instance, argue that a physician's profile should be considered to fall under the routine use exemption because one of the purposes of the PSRO law is to uphold the interests of patients.

It should be noted that even if Privacy Act exemptions are applicable to PSROs to allow disclosure, there may be instances where other legislation will prevent disclosure, such as the exemption provisions of the Freedom of Information Act. Section 1166 of the PSRO law, which authorizes the Secretary to protect privileged PSRO data, may afford adequate protection against disclosure under the Privacy Act. Only litigation will determine whether federal courts in dealing with the Privacy Act will rule that the Secretary's power to exempt PSRO data must be dictated by specific guidelines as is the general rule in the Freedom of Information area.[103]

CONCLUSION

This chapter has tried to provide some background in a complex legal area in which constitutional, regulatory, and common law all have some effect on the protection of peer review data. The discussion of privacy and confidentiality issues in medical peer review focused on six areas: (1) the physician-patient testimonial privilege and independent causes of action for breach of medical confidentiality, (2) the tort of privacy, (3) the constitutional right of privacy, (4) federal legislation dealing with data, the Freedom of Information Act, and the Privacy Act, (5) state information laws, and (6) BQA confidentiality policy for PSROs. These six rather broad and developing legal areas will affect fundamental questions concerning protection of peer review data.

Essentially, the questions with which we are concerned in the privacy and confidentiality areas are easily identifiable: what data should be available, who should have access to it, and what procedures should be implemented for access. Presently, the PSRO program has adequately addressed only the question of access procedures. These data issues are ultimately questions of policy. How that policy shapes the law and develops will depend as much upon public pressure as upon precedents of privacy law. The law as it now stands in the privacy and confidentiality areas is in a fluid state, because there is no national consensus. Until a more crystalized picture of the privacy right emerges, proponents of both full disclosure and no disclosure will be able to draw equally upon the law to support their position. The only safe prognosis we can now make in the area of data protection is that the policies will undergo significant change as public and professional attitudes, the law, and the peer review process itself alter and grow.

NOTES
1. Alan Westin, *Privacy and Freedom* (New York: Atheneum Press, 1967).

2. Arthur Miller, "A Nation of Datamaniacs," *Prism* 2 (1974): 19.

3. Charles Renshaw, "Is Privacy Obsolete?" *Prism* 2 (1974): 13.

4. John Rumsey, "The Patient Trust *Must* Be Protected," *Prism* 2 (1974): 22.

5. Simonsen v. Swenson, 104 Neb. 224, 177 N.W. 831 (1920).

6. Alfred Freedman, "Looking Over the Doctor's Shoulder," *Trial* 11, no. 1 (1975): 28.

7. _____, "PSRO and the Privacy Act: Progress in Confidentiality Guarantees," *Connecticut Medicine* (November 1975): 702.

8. Michael Levett, "Illegal Prying Into Medical Records Told," *Los Angeles Times* (June 12, 1976), p. 1.

9. Abstracting tends to be most accurate where the treatment is clearly defined; it falters in situations where multiple diagnoses are involved.

10. It has been argued that peer review profiles will have little value because they are in a coded form and would not be meaningful to the average consumer without proper interpretation.

11. Insurance companies also assemble large amounts of physician information for payment purposes, but generally the information is not released by the intermediary to the government. Presently, under Titles XVIII and XIX, the information held is of a financial nature. More extensive records have been developed only for physicians investigated for alleged abuses.

12. Charles McCormack, *Law of Evidence* (St. Paul: West Publishing, 1954), p. 213.

13. North Carolina General Statutes §8-53.

14. With the eventual adoption of the Proposed Federal Rules of Evidence, prevention of the disclosure of confidential information may become a legal impossibility.

15. Clark v. Geraci, 208 N.Y.S.2d 564 (1960).

16. Id.

17. The court in the *Hague* case stated that, "A patient should be entitled to freely disclose his symptoms and condition to his doctor in order to receive proper treatment without fear that those facts may become public property.... we conclude, therefore, that ordinarily a physician receives information relating to a patient's health in a confidential capacity and should not disclose such information without the patient's consent, except where the public interest or private interest of the patient so demands." (See 37 N.J. 382, 181 A.2d 345 (1962).)

A Pennsylvania appellate court in *Alexander v. Knight* (197 P. Super. 79, 177 A.2d 142 (1962)), dealing with an unauthorized disclosure problem went one step further. The court condemned a disclosure made prior to trial even though such information would not have been privileged at trial, due to Pennsylvania's lack of physician-patient testimonial privilege. The Pennsylvania court outlined a rigorous fiduciary requirement for physicians to follow: "They owe their patients more than just medical care.... there is a duty of total care: that includes and comprehends a duty to aid the patient in litigation, to render reports when necessary and to attend court when needed. That further includes a duty to refuse affirmative assistance to the patient's antagonist in litigation. The doctor, of course, owes a duty to conscience; to speak the truth he need, however, speak only at the proper time."

18. Simonsen, supra, note 5.

19. Id.

20. Horne v. Patton, 287 S.2d 824 (1974).

21. It is interesting to note that the courts that have strongly supported the confidential relationship between doctor and patient do not view it as an absolute principle, but recognize cases where the trust relationship may be broken, justified by public policy. In *Simonson v. Swenson,* where the physician's disclosure was prompted by a belief, even though incorrect, that it was necessary to prevent disease and his actions were conducted in good faith with reasonable grounds, disclosure was justifiable. In *Hague v. Williams,* the New Jersey court reasoned that where the public interest or private interests of a patient so demand, disclosure may be made to a person with a legitimate interest in the patient's health. Thus, in *Hague v. Williams,* when a physician became aware of a pathological heart condition, he wasn't barred from disclosing such facts to the insurer, for as soon as the parents applied for insurance for their infant child, they lost any rights to nondisclosure they may have possessed. In cases where patients request information from their physicians concerning confidential matters, they often cannot prevent their entire medical history from being divulged. In *Clark v. Geraci* the patient was stopped from challenging his physician's full disclosure of his medical record to the U.S. Air Force, even though the plaintiff requested a partial disclosure.

There are circumstances where a physician may have a duty imposed by law to disclose confidential information concerning his patient in court proceedings for which he cannot be held liable. In *Boyd v. Winn,* 286 Ky. 173, 150 S.W.2d 648 (1941), it was held that a doctor could not be held liable to the patient for divulging privileged information at trial, for, if the doctor did so, he would be held in contempt and subject to penalty. In states where no testimonial privilege exists, it is often the policy to expose medical information when it becomes relevant to the resolution of litigation, thus placing a duty on the physician jurant to do so. While not expressly stated, both parties understand it to be present from either words or conduct. (See Calamari & Perillo, *Contracts,* Sect. 141.)

22. Hammonds v. Aetna Casualty & Surety Company, 243 F. Supp. 793 (1965).

23. Horne, supra, note 20.

24. Clayman v. Bernstein, 30 Pa. D.SC. 543 (1940); Griffin v. Medical Society of New York, 11 N.Y.S.2d 109 (1939).

25. Griswold v. Connecticut, 381 U.S. 479 (1965).

26. Eisenstadt v. Baird, 405 U.S. 438 (1972).

27. Id. at 453.

28. Roe v. Wade, 410 U.S. 113 (1973); Doe v. Bolton, 410 U.S. 179 (1973).

29. Paris Adult Theatre I v. Slaton, 413 U.S. 49 (1973).

30. Doe, supra, note 28.

31. Laird v. Tatum, 408 U.S. 28 (1971).

32. Note, "Right of Privacy," *Northwestern Law Review* 69 (1974): 263, 287.

33. "The Constitution was designed to keep government off the backs of the people. The Bill of Rights was added to keep the precincts of belief, expression of the press, and political and social activities free from surveillance. The Bill of Rights was designed to keep agents of government and official eavesdroppers away from assemblies of the people. The aim was to allow men to be free and independent and to assist their rights against government. There can be no influence more paralyzing of that objective than. . . . surveillance." 408 U.S. 28 (1971). It has been argued that if the Constitutional right of privacy is to protect individual freedom, it must act as a safeguard against an unchecked ability to create massive data banks. While the need for information collection is vital, especially for government medical programs and for health insurance carriers, there is a potential for misuse of the information. It is true that federal legislation provides protection for sensitive

information collected in data banks; but an expansion of the Constitutional privacy doctrine which would limit data collection may ultimately prove a far greater safeguard than legislative protection. If the court is to continue expanding individual privacy rights, it must afford some protection against the abuses inherent in massive data collection.

34. California Bankers Ass'n v. Schultz, 94 S.Ct. 1494 (1974).

35. Freedom of Information Act, 5 USC.

36. Privacy Act, 5 USC 552a.

37. For purposes of the PSRO law, two of these exemptions are important: (B) (6), on medical files, and (B)(3), the statutory exemption section.

38. David Hullet, "Confidentiality of Statistical and Research Data and the Privacy Act of 1974," *Statistical Reporter,* June 1974, p. 197.

39. Barry Boyer, "Computerized Medical Records and the Right to Privacy: The Emerging Federal Response," *Buffalo Law Review* 25 (1975): 37.

40. Privacy Act, §§(f)(1), (f)(5), (d)(1).

41. Federal Register, "OMB Privacy Guidelines," 40 No. 1322 (July 9, 1975), p. 28957.

42. Privacy Act, §§(d)(2), (d)(3).

43. Id. at §(g)(1).

44. Boyer, p. 105.

45. George Annas, "Public Access to Health Care Information," in Gertman and Egdahl, eds., *Quality Assurance in Health Care* (Germantown, Md.: Aspen Systems Corp., 1976).

46. Even without a specific release, disclosing medical records for procurement purposes is considered legitimate.

47. Eric Springer, "PSRO: Some Problems of Confidentiality," *Utah Law Review* (1975): 361, 370, see footnotes 35, 36.

48. Id. See also Charles Jacobs and Susan Weagly, "The Liability Myth Exposed, Hospital Review Activities Pose No Risk," *The PEP Primer* (Chicago: JCAH, 1974).

49. Minn., Second Regular Session Laws, 1974, Ch. 295.

50. Breddice v. Doctors Hospital, 50 F.R.D. 249 D.C. (1970).

51. Id.

52. Jolly v. Superior Court of Pinal County, 540 P.2d 658 (1975).

53. Id. at 662.

54. Matchett v. Superior Court for the County of Yuma, 40 Cal. App.13d 623, 115 *Cal. Rptr.* 317 (1974).

55. Id.

56. Id.

57. Young v. King, Superior Court of New Jersey-Hudson County No. L-16254-73.

58. The Utilization Review Committee is a specific committee, a work of art, so to speak. It is an integral part of the utilization review plan required in order to qualify under the Social Security Act and, thus, participate in federal and state funded programs. The legislature provided special protection to such committees and their members in order to encourage willing participation and, thus, effectively to implement the provisions of Medicare and other health care measures. "Our rules of civil procedure provide for the broadest discovery and any information that may lead to discovery of admissible evidence is discoverable unless privileged. This includes records of hospital committees. . . ." Superior Court of New Jersey-Hudson County, No. L-16254-73.

59. New York Public Officer's Law, §88(2).

60. Freedom of Information Act, supra, note 35.

61. N.Y. Public Officer's Law, supra, note 59.

62. Each agency shall make and publish rules and regulations in conformity with this article, pursuant to such general rules as may be issued by the committee on public access to records, pertaining to availability, location and nature of records. (N.Y. Public Officer's Law §88(2)).

63. In this instance one should be cautioned that state laws cannot be used to access PSRO information which is controlled by federal legislation. In fact, some consumer protection laws specifically exempt entities controlled by federal legislation. (E.g., N.Y. General Business Law §349(d). "In any action it shall be a complete defense that the act or practice is . . . subject to and complies with the rules and regulations of and the statutes administered by . . . any official department, division or agency of the United States.")

64. In some states, the local Freedom of Information Act may block the release of medical review records held by the state. Thus, the attack under consumer protection statutes may only influence access to data held by organizations doing review, such as Foundations for Medical Care and Health Maintenance Organizations.

65. N.Y. General Business Law, §349(a).

66. Mass. General Laws, Ch. 93a, §1.

67. Harvard Center for Community Health, *PSRO Information and Consumer Choice: The Case for Public Disclosure of Health Services Data* (Boston: Harvard Center for Community Health, 1975).

68. Id.

69. Such argument of applying consumer protection laws to peer review committees may be defeated in some states by protective statutes preventing release of medical committee records.

70. The need of the consumer may, in fact, eventually be felt by courts to outweigh the need for confidentiality in the peer review process, especially when the nature and format in which the information will appear is better understood.

71. Some state courts may not be as liberal as Massachusetts, but may require a showing of damages to the consumer of a measurable dollar amount.

72. Commonwealth v. DeCotis, 316 N.E.2d 748 (1974).

73. Id.

74. Id.

75. P.L. 92-603, §116, 42 USC §1320c-15(b).

76. Release of physician profiles may, in fact, be a desirable alternative to sanction; the thought being that the possibility of making practice information public where serious deviation has occurred will act as an incentive for the practitioner to conform to peer review standards of practice.

77. Interim confidentiality regulations allow for the disclosure of data which has been published, which has not been identified by the source of the data and information as confidential, and whose disclosure is not prohibited by law. A PSRO shall also disclose UHDDS data provided it doesn't identify an individual patient or practitioner. In the case of an institution where only one surgeon performs a given type of surgery, release of aggregate data would be directly identifiable to that individual, thus not all UHDDS data will be subject to release.

78. DHW, PSRO Transmittal Letter No. 16, 1975, portions suspended by transmittal No. 41, October 1976; see also Interim Confidentiality Regulations, F.R. v. 41, no. 234 (December 3, 197—): 532.5.

79. While institutional information may eventually not be privileged, manpower limitations may require the PSRO to depend on an area hospital to collect requested information about itself, thus having a potential effect on the type of information released.

80. DHEW, *Guidelines for Implementation of the DHEW-PSRO Confidentiality Policy* (Washington, D.C.: BQA, March 1976). The federal confidentiality policy outlined in Transmittal 16 has been altered with the issuance of Transmittal 41 (October 6, 1976). Pressure of threatened litigation forced BQA to reassess its confidentiality policy. Chances are, however, that once regulations now being developed are issued, they will be similar to Transmittal 16. The PSRO statute itself does not provide BQA with the flexibility of operation in the confidentiality area as was originally felt; issuance of regulation may alter that. Witness changes made by Interim Regulations, December 3, in response to HSA needs.

81. When a physician is sanctioned, copies of the sanction report are sent to the state licensing board, but the physician involved must be notified 15 days prior to disclosure to permit an accompanying statement to be submitted to the licensing board. Copies of privileged information concerning physicians and institutions can be made available to those identifiable parties, but not to patients, who only have the right to inspect their records.

82. Whether such a profile could be admitted into evidence at trial is a matter to be discussed in Chapter 7.

83. Whether an individual can request his/her own PSRO record for use at trial has yet to be tested.

84. It shall be unlawful for any person to disclose such information other than for such purposes, and any person violating the provisions of this section shall, upon conviction, "be fined not more than $1,000, and imprisoned for not more than six months, or both, together with the cost of prosecution." (§1166(B)).

85. Confidentiality Guidelines, supra, note 80 at 44.

86. Transmittal No. 16, supra, note 78 at no. 26.

87. Id.

88. Exemptions in the act may provide adequate protection against such occurrence.

89. The legal status of a PSRO can only be settled through litigation in federal court and thus neither the private corporation nor the agency theory can be ruled out. See Chapter 5.

90. P.L. 93-502.

91. This method of assessing an exemption by measuring the need to know with the type and extent of the personal invasion is unique to this exemption (Getman v. NLRB).

92. Note, "Freedom of Information Act Assessment," *Columbia Law Review* 74 (1974): 896, 953.

93. Regulations have the same legal effect as statutes; both are law.

94. Vaughn v. Rosen, 484 F.2d 820 (1973).

95. Stretch v. Weinberger, 495 F.2d 639 (1974).

96. The legislative history of this section so indicates.

97. It is clear in reading the draft guidelines that BQA attempted to follow the dictates of the Privacy Act as closely as possible. For example, in Transmittal 16 there was no men-

tion of special procedure for minors to access their records, but the draft guidelines set up such a procedure as required under the Privacy Act.

98. Confidentiality Guidelines, p. 3 (April 1976, draft).

99. While the Secretary of HEW may determine agency policy as to whether the Privacy Act should be extended to government contractors, one could challenge the decision in court, holding that there is no rational basis for excluding PSROs while applying the Act to fiscal intermediaries. Before a court would uphold the Secretary's position not to apply the Privacy Act to PSROs, it would have to be convinced of the fact that PRSOs' operational functions were not as closely tied into a function of Medicare and Medicaid as the fiscal intermediary. See also Senate Finance Comm. Report No. 92-1230, p. 69.

100. Boyer, supra, note 39; see also 40 Fed. Reg. 47406.

101. Sen. Fin. Comm. Rept. (92-1230), p. 44.

102. 40 Fed. Reg. 47408. In order for the Freedom of Information Act exemption to be relevant to PSROs, it would first have to be demonstrated that the act applies. For the court order exemption to apply, the Secretary's ban on the court subpoena of PSRO data would have to be overcome.

103. Id. The legislative history of the Privacy Act indicates that the exceptions under the Act are not to be subject to a balancing of interest approach, as was the case under the Freedom of Information Act. "The Privacy Act . . . adopted a blanket approach that confers on the data subject control over the dissemination of all records [with certain rigid exceptions] without reference to the nature of the information they contain." (*Michigan Law Review* 73, nos. 6 & 7 (1975): 1337). If the Privacy Act applies to the PSRO, use of Social Security numbers may be limited. Section 7 of the Privacy Act makes use of a Social Security number voluntary (unless the PSRO statute were amended to make such disclosure mandatory). The agency requiring the disclosure must also inform the individual how the Social Security number will be used.

Chapter 7

Peer Review and Medical Malpractice

Medical malpractice law is currently undergoing widespread changes caused by severe pressure placed upon the present tort system as a result of the increase in claims and a concomitant rise in rates of liability insurance coverage. The changes suggested, and in some cases implemented, in response to the concerns of organized medicine range from arbitration panels to limitations on awards and attorneys' fees.

The debate surrounding medical malpractice has done little to aid the climate in which medicine is practiced. The liability issue has apparently become a concern of foremost importance in the minds of physicians, health professionals and administrators of medical institutions alike. From the public standpoint, many of the safeguards physicians are taking against liability are desirable. But some professionals look upon the safeguards as "defensive medicine," and many lawyers think that the climate of fear has led to distortions in physicians' understanding of the real risks of medical liability. While new medical procedures and techniques raise serious concerns about potential effects upon malpractice liability, the implementation of peer review has engendered concern about the possible effect it may have on the medical liability problem.

The issue of malpractice and the peer review process may, in fact, pose few potential difficulties. Various statutory provisions exist, as discussed, which protect peer review committee records from being used in a state or federal court. Immunity laws isolate committee members from liability in their role as reviewers. It seems that the present "due care" standard will not be altered as a result of peer review committee procedures, as seen in the terms of the PSRO law. We cannot, however, overlook the fact that peer review committees and their members may become embroiled in medical malpractice problems. Legislation may act

163

as a protection against less than the full range of liability problems. For example, individual peer review committee records may not be used in court, but what about the evaluative tools (norms, standards, criteria) developed by physicians to judge their peers' behavior? Will these be usable in a negligence action? Certainly, it would seem that peer review norms, standards and criteria representing a consensus of medical opinion may eventually be introduced and accepted as evidence in malpractice cases.[1]

The purpose of this chapter is to evaluate the potential effect the peer review process may have on medical malpractice. The chapter will develop some background material on medical negligence; discuss the impact of the immunity provision in §1167 of the PSRO law as it affects the "due care" standard; consider the question of admissibility of peer review guidelines and records as evidence in a malpractice trial: and conclude with a consideration of how peer review could affect medical negligence if used as a method of legal arbitration and as a corrective educational device. It must be remembered that the relationship of medical malpractice and peer review is at present of a speculative nature, and that long-term predictions about what will occur are difficult in view of changes that may take place in both areas.

MEDICAL MALPRACTICE LAW BACKGROUND

Medical malpractice has been defined as "a particular form of negligence that consists of not applying to the exercise of the practice of medicine that degree of care and skill which is ordinarily employed by the profession generally under similar conditions and in like surrounding circumstances." [2] Another common definition of malpractice is that it is "negligence that consists of not applying to the exercise of the practice of medicine that degree of care and skill which is ordinarily applied by the profession generally under similar conditions and in like surroundings." [3]

Medical malpractice has been characterized as having four key elements: "(1) the failure of the physician in the treatment of a patient to possess and employ that reasonable degree of learning, skill, and experience which is ordinarily possessed by others of his profession, (2) the failure to exercise reasonable and ordinary care and diligence in the performance of the physician's skill and application of knowledge, (3) failure to exert proper judgment in a given case, (4) the failure to demonstrate the skill and capacity of other physicians in the same specialty in a similar environment." [4]

The medical negligence case is basically similar to other liability actions in that the plaintiff must demonstrate three basic elements: Breach of a duty owed, proximate cause, and damage. There first must be a showing of duty existing between the plaintiff patient and defendant physician. The duty owed to the patient by the physician is established by the treatment relationship, and generally the existence of such relationship is not an issue.[5] The key element required in most medical malpractice cases is a showing that the act or omission of the defendant physician was the proximate or legal cause of the injury to the plaintiff. Even if a patient can prove that a physician or surgeon did not meet the required standard of care, he cannot recover damages unless he can also prove that the negligence caused him injuries which would not have occurred in its absence.[6] Finally, damages (compensatory and punitive) suffered by the plaintiff must be proved, for the negligence action exists to compensate measurable injury; without a showing of injury, liability has little significance.

A physician is held to the standard of "due care," which means that in any given case, the individual must exercise appropriate professional judgment (use of adequate knowledge and skill in the treatment of a patient).

The "due care" standard is the underlying measurement in determining whether a practitioner's behavior in a given case was acceptable. What is considered "due care" is variable, in view of the fact that the standard fluctuates with the physician, the patient, and the situation in which treatment was delivered. For instance, what is considered acceptable behavior in a medical emergency occurring outside a hospital is quite different from what is considered reasonable behavior in a hospital emergency room. Similarly, the standard of care applied to a general practitioner may not be the same as that applied to a specialist in an identical situation.[7]

In the process of evaluating whether or not a physician defendant exercised "due care" in a given situation, a number of factors come into play. The defendant's training, specialty and locality of practice are all factors that courts consider in determining the standard to be applied to the defendant physician.

At trial a jury may rely on the testimony of a medical expert in evaluating whether a physician has acted reasonably in a given case. The expert witness has a dual function in testifying: the first is to define the acceptable professional standards relevant to the case at hand, the second is to express an opinion concerning the cause of the injury being litigated. The expert can express an opinion on the causative factor, but generally cannot testify that the defendant was in fact negligent.[8]

Until recently, physicians were judged by what their peers in the community or similar community would do in a given situation. Due care was thus measured, and evaluated by the expert, on the basis of the recognized norm of practice in a given community. More recently, in most jurisdictions the locality approach to evaluating physician behavior has been abrogated; the local standard is seen as only one factor to be considered in assessing due care.[9]

Generally, physicians are now judged on the basis of national standards developed as a result of a consensus by practitioners throughout the country. This national approach was first seen in cases involving medical specialties, where it became evident that those claiming themselves as uniquely qualified in a given area quite often had no local basis of comparison and, thus, had to be evaluated on the basis of what similar specialists in other localities considered acceptable practice.[10]

IMMUNITY AND DUE CARE

The Senate Finance Committee stated that "the intention [of §1167] is to remove any inhibition to proper exercise of PSRO functions, or the following, by practitioners and providers, of standards and norms recommended by the review organization." [11] However, the law on its face can be read only as requiring what the common law already requires. As it stands, §1167 appears merely to reiterate due care standards presently applied by the common law. The section states that even if a physician follows the PSRO review guidelines, he will "gain" immunity from malpractice liability only if he also has exercised "due care" in the treatment rendered.[12] Thus, a physician sued for malpractice cannot escape liability via the immunity clause by pleading compliance with PSRO norms, standards, and/or criteria unless proof of compliance is accompanied by a showing of professional due care and diligence.[13]

The immunity section, while not supplanting the due care standard, may nevertheless be significant in some malpractice actions. Basically, malpractice actions can be classified as involving errors in either treatment or diagnosis with treatment split further into errors of skill or methodology. In a malpractice case based on the defendant's alleged negligence in selecting an incorrect method of treatment, the use of a PSRO criterion or standard may have strong evidentiary value. A violation of a PSRO standard, which can be interpreted as deviation from an acceptable range of behavior, may in some instances be a strong indication of improper professional behavior. Failure to conform to specific treatment elements may be medically and legally justified because a given case may require certain treatment procedures not specifically listed by the PSRO; criteria lists are not "cookbooks" but rather evaluative tools subject to alteration. Violation of a norm ought not in and of itself be very strong evidence of negligence, especially in any unusual set of circumstances. Apparently agreeing, the Senate Finance Committee report stated, "Failure to order or provide care in accordance with the norms employed by PSRO is not intended to create a legal presumption of liability." [14]

Nevertheless, if a court allows the PSRO standard into evidence, such information may be helpful in evaluating the conduct of the allegedly negligent physician. A demonstration that the physician being sued acted in accordance with PSRO standards may help prove that adequate skill and diligence were exercised. This is not to say that the conformance to or violation of a PSRO standard would by itself constitute or refute negligence, for a showing of "due care" would still be required. However, a jury of twelve non-physicians can be expected to give strong weight to an impartial standard developed by physicians for nonadversary uses. The PSRO standard may in some cases have a very positive effect for the defendant, which is what the framers of §1167 intended. In fact, the *Finance Committee Report* indicates that Congress intended that the PSRO review guidelines could be used to defend during negligence lawsuits. However, once a PSRO guideline is introduced in court, both parties can draw upon it equally for affirmative or defensive purposes. Furthermore, the Senate's hope that guidelines would be used only in defense is not binding on state or federal courts, as it is not part of the statute itself. It might well, in fact, be a denial of due process for Congress to design a mechanism which generates information that cannot be used equally by both parties to a litigation.

ADMISSIBILITY

Peer Review Guidelines

In evaluating the impact that PSRO and other peer review program guidelines will have on medical malpractice, we must first look at the guidelines' impact on malpractice law. The question of the guidelines' admissibility as evidence at trial is crucial in determining the overall effect the review process will have on medical negligence law.

Certain objections may be raised at trial which will prevent PSRO guidelines, or records and documents, from being introduced into evidence. Introduction of PSRO information could be challenged on the basis of several objections: hearsay, physician-patient privilege, best evidence, inability to use past performance to demonstrate negligence, or relevance.

Hearsay

Hearsay evidence is any out-of-court writing or statement that is offered in court to prove the truth of some event or assertion; generally, unless such evidence falls under a specific "exception," it will not be admissable.[15] The legal presumption of nonadmissibility is called the hearsay rule. The hearsay rule does not apply to hearsay which is covered by a specific exception in the rules of evidence. In addition, some courts are governed by rules of evidence which permit them to allow any hearsay into evidence if it can be demonstrated that the hearsay statement is reliable and necessary for the proof of the case at hand. In assessing reliability of information, a court will consider its relevancy and accuracy.[16]

It would seem initially that PSRO norms, standards, and criteria would be barred from use in malpractice cases on the grounds that the standards are hearsay evidence. Peer review guidelines would fall under the hearsay category as material developed out of court which is brought into evidence in the attempt to prove the truth of one of the litigants' positions. To demonstrate to a court the reasons why peer review guidelines should be used, such material would have to be shown to be both trustworthy and necessary to a malpractice litigation. Counsel attempting to introduce PSRO review guidelines into evidence would have to demonstrate how review guidelines were made, why they represent a consensus of medical opinion, what flexibility there is in applying the measures of evaluations, and what relevancy the guidelines have as proof.

In order to provide adequate information to a court concerning review guidelines, a physician on the criteria committee (preferably the chairman of the audit committee) might have to testify on how peer review guidelines are developed. Other medical experts in the involved specialty might have to testify to verify the fact that PSRO evaluative measures represent a consensus of professional opinion. Without a proper foundation, most courts will not admit peer review guidelines as evidence. After a period of time during which peer review norms, standards, and criteria are increasingly used in litigation, judicial recognition may eventually be awarded these guidelines so that they will be subject only to the test of relevancy, and not questioned as to trustworthiness and acceptability.

A parallel can be drawn between the admissibility of peer review committee norms, standards, and criteria, and the admission of medical texts into evidence. Many American jurisdictions prohibit the introduction of medical texts directly into evidence, and allow them only for a limited purpose on cross-examination. In fact, use of medical texts on cross-examination is probably less limited than theory indicates, but if referred to on direct examination, these texts are often powerful evidence in establishing the standard of care.[17]

Persuasive arguments designed to overcome hearsay objections have been made about the reliability of medical textbooks. The Supreme Court of Wisconsin, in the case of *Halladin v. Peterson,* ruled that a plaintiff in a medical malpractice action may establish the standard of care and breach of that standard by use of medical texts.[18] There is a demonstrable trend toward greater use of medical treatises as evidence in their own right, as can be seen in both the Uniform Rules of Evidence and the Proposed Rule of Evidence for U.S. District Courts. Such a trend creates a more favorable climate in which to explore the possibility of admitting peer review guidelines into evidence.[19]

While peer review committee guidelines are not identical to medical texts for evidentiary purposes, the two are similar because both will usually be introduced to demonstrate acceptable professional behavior. Either party at trial will be able to draw upon peer review guidelines like medical texts and use those guidelines for supportive or rebuttal purposes.

Relevance

Another bar against the admissibility of peer review guidelines in negligence lawsuits is the question of whether these guidelines are applicable in all medical cases. In other words, do PSRO or other review group evaluative measures only apply in cases involving patients reviewed by the respective programs (Title V, XVIII, XIX patients), or will they apply generally to everyone? It would seem, at least initially, that courts might be rather "strict," admitting peer review guidelines only where they apply directly to the individual litigant. While initially the applicability of guidelines may be limited, it is reasonable to assume that medical practice guidelines, locally developed and reflective of acceptable treatment, will ultimately be applied by courts beyond the programs for which they were specifically created.

In General

It has been suggested that use of peer review guidelines in malpractice actions would constitute a return to the locality rule: i.e., medical care will again be judged by what is done in the local area where suit is brought, and not by national medical standards, as is the current trend. If each PSRO or peer review committee can develop its norms, standards, and criteria locally, these measures of evaluation may vary from region to region. While some variation may be present, generally the norms, standards, and criteria used by peer review groups will be quite similar.[20] For instance, the sources for criteria are often obtained from national services (AMA criteria lists); locally developed criteria have not yet demonstrated great variation. The differences in medical practice from area to area seem to be centered in length of stay and cost, rather than the type of medical treatment followed in any given area. However, this lack of variability may merely reflect that the primary emphasis of most local groups' review so far has been length of stay.

While use of peer review guidelines can have a definite evidentiary effect in a malpractice case, it is probable that these guidelines will not significantly affect the outcome of most medical negligence suits. The norms, standards, and criteria used by peer review committees will be of a general nature; that is, they will allow for a reasonable degree of variability and will permit a major variance if medically justified. If behavior so deviates from peer review guidelines as to border on negligence, this fact may be clear to a jury, irrespective of the use of peer review guidelines. In most malpractice cases, the issue of negligence is not clear-cut; therefore, the peer review guidelines will not usually be adequate to demonstrate liability or the lack of it. Generally, expert witnesses will still be required to demonstrate whether, in their opinion, the defendant lived up to the standards of acceptable medical practice.

PSRO Records and Documents

In examining the question of admissibility, we are concerned not only with the admission into evidence of PSRO review guidelines, but also with the admission of peer review committee records and notes.[21]

Statutory Protections

To be fully effective, the BQA policy which prohibits the admission of PSRO material into evidence would have to be determined by courts to take precedence over state law.

Some states have enacted statutes designed to prevent the subpoena and discovery of peer review committee records, or at least classify such records as "privileged," thus preventing their admission into evidence. These state laws remain for the most part untested.[22] In jurisdictions with special protective legislation for medical committee documents,

PSRO records (federal policy aside) will probably be inadmissible.[23] In states with no legislation dealing with peer review committee records, or very weak legislation, PSROs would have to rely on the "federal preemption" doctrine. If it is determined that a state law "stands as an obstacle to the accomplishment and execution of the full purposes and objectives of Congress," then that law is superseded by the federal law.[24]

In raising an objection to introduction of privileged PSRO records, a state court's attention would not only have to be directed to any existing conflict between federal and state law, but, more importantly, to the rationale underlying the policy for PSRO record confidentiality. The most likely result would be that state courts would recognize the privileged nature of PSRO information and neither allow it to be admitted into evidence nor allow its use for discovery purposes. PSRO information that is not privileged (institutional data or information not recognized as being privileged in a state court) may possibly be inadmissable for other reasons.[25]

Finally, in considering the question of admissibility of nonPSRO peer review committee records, the effect of protective state legislation must be considered.[26] Some of the state laws which prevent the discovery of peer review records also prevent their admission into evidence. In those jurisdictions which legislatively bar admissability of peer review committee records, such statutes would act conclusively to protect all medical review records from being used in court.[27] Presumably, even if peer review committee records are not covered by nonadmissibility provisions, in states granting such information "privileged" status, admission would be barred.

State courts are generally rather "strict" in interpreting nonadmissibility statutes, and will not expand protection to matter not specifically listed. In *Tucson Medical Center v. Misvech*[28] the Arizona Supreme Court addressed the question of admissibility of evidence stemming from medical committee review. Arizona has a statute which prevents the admissibility of medical review committee records into evidence. The court distinguished committee records from minutes or evidence considered by the committee, and held the latter to be subject to a limited form of subpoena. The Arizona Court said that, "Statements and information considered by the medical peer review committee are subject to subpoena for the determination of the trial judge," as to whether they will be admissible in evidence.

The Physician-Patient Privilege

Introduction into evidence of a patient profile could be challenged on the basis that it violates the physician-patient privilege. The privilege, as was discussed in the chapter on confidentiality, allows the patient to prevent the admission of information developed in the course of the treatment relationship. In order to admit a PSRO patient profile into evidence, the identifiable patient may have to give permission before this data can be used in court. This privilege, however, is a weak one; and as was discussed in Chapter 6, it is often up to the court's discretion as to whether patient data should be admitted.

Best Evidence

The best evidence rule (also referred to as the "original documents rule") requires the production of primary source evidence.[29] PSRO documents are constructed from abstracts of medical records and are, at best, a secondary source of information. There are, however, cases where physician or institutional practice patterns will be relevant, and so profiles in such an instance may become primary sources of information (e.g., licensure revocations, or lawsuits in which a hospital is charged with failure to take corrective action to prevent alleged negligence).

Hearsay: Records and Reliability

Records of any kind are generally judged to be hearsay evidence and must qualify for admission at trial under some exception to the hearsay rule. The most clearly applicable is the business records exception. This exception allows records to be introduced into evidence provided that: (1) the custodian or other qualified witness testifies concerning their identity and mode of preparation, and (2) it can be shown that the source of information was accurate and the document was made in the regular course of business.[30]

An article in the *University of California at Davis Law Review* argued that physician[31] and institutional profiles fulfill most of the requirements delineated under the business records exception: "These are: (1) the computer profile printout is made in the regular course of business, (2) the source of the information and method of preparation are trustworthy, and (3) a custodian or other qualified witness will be able to testify as to its identity and mode of preparation."[32]

While it may be theoretically desirable to use physician and institutional profiles in court proceedings to determine patterns of behavior, there are serious questions about the accuracy of certain types of profiles. A physician profile is based on "abstracts" of records, and abstracting techniques are still in a developmental stage. For example, a very basic problem in abstracting medical cases with multiple diagnoses is that in many situations it is difficult or impossible for the abstractor to identify the primary diagnosis, and the resulting errors reduce the reliability of profiles. Another basic difficulty in abstracting is that the medical record, the primary source of data, tends in some cases to be incomplete, inaccurate, or unreadable.

The current problems with abstracting methodology place the question of admitting medical profiles into evidence in doubt. While certain types of profiles may be quite accurate (e.g., in such areas as surgery), other medical and psychiatric profiles may be less trustworthy. Admissibility of profile evidence would require a court to evaluate the type of profile being introduced, as to whether a sufficient degree of accuracy was present.

It should be noted that, while state courts may not presently allow profiles to be admitted into evidence, in the absence of specific protective legislation they may allow "discovery" of such profiles for trial preparation purposes. Also, physicians' profiles may be admissible at administrative hearings, where the rules of evidence are usually more flexible than at judicial trials. For example, a profile that presents a picture of a physician's behavior over a given period of time may be valuable information used by a committee in a licensure revocation hearing. An argument in favor of such use is that all the panel members would likely be adequately acquainted with medical profiles, so that the chances of misinterpretation would not be as real as in a judicial forum.

Other types of records held by a PSRO or peer review committee are likely to be held inadmissible, such as sanction reports, notes on the committee's deliberations about a practitioner, etc. Although one could argue that such PSRO committee notes fit the definition of an admissible business record (i.e., that they were made in the regular course of business at the time of the meeting and are verifiable),[33] it is probable that such data would be viewed as composed of evidence of past performances, and therefore could not be used to show negligence.[34]

Profiles and the Past Performance Rule

The law of evidence prevents the use of past performance as a means of demonstrating negligence in a specific instance.[35]

Anyone who attempts to admit a physician's profile into a court proceeding would have to overcome the rule of evidence that prohibits the use of a person's character to prove conduct circumstantially: "Where a negligent act by the defendant or his servant is an issue most courts will reject proof of the actor's reputation for care or negligence."[36] Even if a physician's peer review profile clearly demonstrated a poor record of performances in past cases, one could not introduce it into evidence to show that the defendant physician committed malpractice in the litigated case.

But the rule of exclusion is not absolute. For instance, character evidence can be used to establish motive, intent, purpose, etc.[37] In *Gonzales v. Nork*, where the question of malpractice insurance payment was at issue, evidence of approximately 50 other medical cases was introduced to, "show (1) the intent of the defendant doctor to commit fraud, and (2) knowledge of the hospital authorities about that fraud. While computer profile evidence was not used in Nork, statistical analysis of what the defendant doctor had done in a series of similar cases was used, and similar principles are involved in use of computer profile evidence."[38]

Use of institutional profiles may be quite helpful in malpractice suits in which the hospital or other health facility is being held corporately liable for a negligent occurrence. The institutional profile in and of itself will not prove malpractice or its absence, but it may be valuable evidence in demonstrating a high or low rate of occurrence of certain procedures in the institution. The objection about past performance not being relevant to show present negligence discussed above would hold for institutional profiles; but chances are that such evidence would be introduced to demonstrate a pattern of behavior that indicates the institution's failure to take corrective action about a continuing problem as opposed to a specific incident of negligence.

The argument against admitting evidence of past performance to prove negligence is not, one should note, applicable to licensure proceedings (e.g., suspension or revocation), where it is the totality of past behavior, rather than a single instance of negligence, that is the reason for the proceeding. In such licensure cases, physicians' profiles could prove to be the most useful evidence available. As the California law review article noted, "In many cases, the negligence becomes visible only when the totality of the doctor's behavior can be considered—that is, when his overall performance in the plaintiff's and all similar cases can be evaluated."[39]

ALTERNATIVE USES OF PEER REVIEW

Malpractice Arbiter

It has been suggested that peer review groups be used as screening panels for medical malpractice cases. In light of the pressure placed upon the judicial system as a result of the medical malpractice crisis, the idea of using medical panels to judge negligence issues promises possible cost and time savings. It also may create a more precise alternative fact-finding and decision-making process. The peer review committee would be able to base its evaluation on guidelines arguably more precise than those used by juries and nonphysician judges. Under most pretrial screening proposals, the reviewers are not actually able to declare their colleague legally liable, but their findings are admissable, and if negative would presumably establish a strong presumption of liability in court.

Use of peer review groups to act as arbiters of medical negligence actions would significantly alter the medical review system. The determinations now made by peer review panels deal with questions of medical cost and quality, not with legal liability. The fact that a practitioner receives a denial from a physician review committee, or that his request for admission certification is rejected by an appeals committee, doesn't indicate that he is guilty of malpractice. Even the physician who is actually sanctioned by a medical review group may not be negligent.[40] Denial, and more particularly peer review sanction, should indicate an error or errors in medical judgment and practice, but to equate that with the commission of a legally compensable wrong would be incorrect.

Making medical review function as legal review would cause the entire process to become less open. Review committees would adopt a defensive posture and would, like state licensure boards, become reluctant to make adverse decisions or recommendations except in extreme circumstances. Informality in committee deliberations would be lost and the intermediate sanctions of consultation and compromise with the deviant practitioner would tend to become less feasible. Making PSROs responsible as a legal arbiter would change the nature of the organization and make the establishment of relations with area physicians extremely difficult.

Educational Force

Peer review may prove to be a valuable educational tool to prevent malpractice or poor practice. Peer review can highlight professional deficiencies in a practitioner's behavior, and the profile developed from review could give a physician some indication of areas in which he needs improvement. It has been suggested that whenever peer review finds deficiencies, those physicians involved should be advised to take continuing medical education courses in areas in which they are demonstrated to be weak. While there is no established correlation between the incidence of medical negligence lawsuits and the badness of practitioners, it is possible that medical practice could be positively affected by identifying problem areas and providing education in those areas. It has even been suggested that peer review committee findings of deficiencies could be turned over to state licensing boards, which, if given authority under law, could require certain physicians to undergo further training.

CONCLUSION

Will peer review programs increase or decrease the incidence of medical malpractice? It is difficult to assess the ultimate impact of peer review on medical negligence in view of the developments in both areas. Initially, it would seem that a decision by a peer review organization to deny admission or continued stay may make worse a poor physician-patient relationship. The denial may act as a red flag, demonstrating to a patient that his physician had done something wrong. If a denial is not adequately explained by the physician, the patient may decide to pursue legal action if he feels the denial was unjust. Clearly, the patient will have to be carefully informed of his right to an appeal by both the PSRO and the attending physician; and, in some cases, the physician may feel it necessary to pursue an appeal on behalf of the patient.

Generally, it can be presumed that the physician admits a patient in good faith without knowing that there will be a denial of that particular admission. Even if the physician realizes that a given admission may be questionable, he is usually not personally liable for the financial loss to the patient resulting from the denial; and if there is potential liability, it is hard to prove that the financial or other harm flowed from the admission.

Peer review denials may therefore lead to an increase in the incidence of lawsuits, but not necessarily the incidence of findings of negligence. If this happens, however, it could place an added strain on court systems that are already having problems handling current caseloads.

On the other hand, if peer review is successful in educating physicians to ways of improving their behavior, it may have the effect of upgrading medical practice. While it is true, as previously stated, that malpractice suits and poor practice are not always synonymous, reduction in unnecessary hospitalization and improvement in practice procedures could possibly have a positive effect on the liability problem. Thus, if successful peer review can effectuate positive change in medical behavior, it may act to reduce the incidence of negligence and negligence claims.

NOTES

1. Use of the peer review process itself has been suggested as a potential screening device for malpractice cases, a usage that may prove to frustrate and abuse the entire process.

2. Prosser, *Torts* (St. Paul: West, 1971), Ch. 5 §32.

3. "Physicians & Surgeons," *Am. Jur.* 2d, §110.

4. American Law Institute, *Restatement of the Law of Torts* (St. Paul: West), §457 (1965).

5. Angela Holder, *Medical Malpractice Law*, New York: Wiley & Sons, 1975, Chapt. 2.

6. Such a relationship has created the legal notion of "quasi-contract" existing between the parties. On the basis of this quasi-contractual relationship, physicians who violate the inherent terms of the agreement (e.g., not holding communications in confidence), have been sued on a breach-of-contract theory. Generally, only in cases where a physician is being held liable for actions of a third party (the so-called "captain of the ship" doctrine) does the question of the scope of the defendant's duty become an important concern.

7. While the general practitioner is held to the standard of care of "the reasonable careful and prudent physician," in most jurisdictions a specialist is required to adhere to the standard of the "reasonable careful and prudent specialist in his field." A specialist is one who has a "special degree of skill and care which physicians similarly situated who devote special study and attention to the treatment of such organ, disease, or injury ordinarily possess." The type of care the law requires to be exercised by physicians varies: Both G.P.s and specialists have unique responsibilities in the same case. The specialist may be held to a higher standard of care, but the G.P. may be liable for failure to seek consultation or refer the case to another physician.

8. Expert testimony is essential in malpractice cases in which the plaintiff must rely on members of the defendant's profession to prove the standard of care or skill ordinarily used in the practice of that profession at a particular place, since they alone know such standards. There are instances in which it is not required to prove malpractice, but generally expert testimony is essential to a showing of medical negligence. The cause of the injury and the acceptable medical standard are often interrelated issues, in that selection of appropriate treatment methods may have prevented the injury. This, of course, is not always true. There are cases in which, even if the appropriate medical procedures were followed, the defendant could have performed the procedure in a negligent fashion.

9. The locality rule has no present validity except that it may be considered one of the elements to determine the degree of care and skill expected of the average practitioner of the class to which he belongs. No longer is it proper to limit the definition of the standard of care which a medical doctor or dentist must meet solely to the practice or custom of a particular locality, a similar locality, or a geographical area.

10. An alternative way of demonstrating negligence other than by a showing of lack of due care is by use of the evidentiary principle of *res ipsa loquitur.* If successfully demonstrated, this principle creates an inference of negligence, shifting the burden of proof to the defendant to counter the inference. The doctrine requires three elements in order for it to apply: "(1) The event is the kind which ordinarily does not occur in the absence of negligence; (2) other responsible causes, including the conduct of the plaintiff and third persons, are sufficiently eliminated by the evidence; and (3) the indicated negligence is within the scope of the defendant's duty to the plaintiff." The classic *res ipsa loquitur* case involves a situation where there is a noninherent risk involved in carrying out a certain procedure and injury results (i.e. injury could not have occurred unless there was a lack of due care). In the more common malpractice case, the risk is inherent in the proce-

dure performed; thus a demonstration of injury is not enough to utilize the *res ipsa doctrine:* A showing of negligent conduct must generally be included.

11. Report of the Senate Finance Committee, No. 92-1230, p. 267.

12. P.L.92-603, §1167, 42 USC §1320-15(c).

13. For the purposes of this chapter, the terms norms, standards, and criteria will be referred to collectively as PSRO evaluative measures or as peer review guidelines. One should be cautioned in not confusing the standard used by a peer review organization with a legal standard, for the former only represents a medical judgment.

14. Senate Finance Committee Report, p. 267.

15. Charles McCormack, *The Law of Evidence* (St. Paul: West, 1954), §195.

16. Federal Rules of Evidence for U.S. District Courts, Rule 803 (24), 1975 ed.

17. One should not be confused by the use of texts by experts on direct examination to support their position; this is not the same thing as introducing these treaties directly into evidence, although a jury may not appreciate this distinction.

18. Halladin v. Peterson, 39 Wisc.2d 668, 159 N.W.2d 738 (1968).

19. *The Uniform Rules of Evidence* permits the use of any reliable published authority to prove the truth of the matter stated as an exception to the heresay rule. The *Federal Rules of Evidence for the U.S. District Courts* provides for the admission of medical books "to the extent called to the attention of an expert witness upon cross examination or relied upon by him in direct examination, statements contained in published treaties, periodicals, or pamphlets on a subject of medicine . . . established as a reliable authority by the testimony or admission of the witness or by other expert testimony or by judicial notice." (Rule 803 (18) FRE 1975).

20. For most diagnostic categories, the peer review guidelines would merely reflect acceptable practice in a given area, and wide use of peer review guidelines may in fact tend to upgrade practice standards in some areas.

21. While the question of discovery of peer review records (covered in Chapter 6) is related to the issue of admissibility of evidence, the two areas are of separate concern. Admissibility of evidence means that, in this case, PSRO or other peer review committee records and documents can be formally admitted as evidence in a trial, and that therefore, such material can be used as proof to substantiate one's position (which can be referred to as groundwork upon which to develop other evidence). Discovery allows one to examine records in preparation for trial, but such examination does not necessarily mean that the discovered material can be admitted into evidence.

22. Eric Springer, "Professional Standards Review Organizations: Some Problems of Confidentiality," 2 *Utah Law Review* 365 (1975).

23. Charles Jacobs, and Susan Weagly, *The PEP Primer* (Chicago: JCAH, 1974).

24. U.S. Constitution, Article VII §2.

25. The authors believe that most state courts will uphold federal policy on confidentiality of medical records even if they do not have special state laws. However, there is a chance that state courts will not recognize federal policy on this matter, as in certain instances they may feel that peer review reports are crucial to the resolution of a given dispute. We must, therefore, be concerned with other exclusionary methods relevant to protecting information. The discussion in this section will pertain not only to PSRO records, but also to those state and private peer review committee records that are not covered by some type of protective legislation.

26. One should not rely on state statutes to prohibit discovery and/or admissibility of peer review committee records, because of the variability of such statutes in application. While some state laws are comprehensive, in that they form a conclusive protection against admissibility, others do not. Traditional rules of evidence may have to be invoked to prohibit peer review committee records from trial in states which do not provide extensive protection.

27. Jacobs and Weagly.

28. *Tucson Medical Center v. Misvech,* 545 P.2d 958, 113 Ariz. 34 (1976).

29. McCormick, supra, note 15, §195.

30. Hospital records do not technically fall within the business record exception but have been admitted under special statutory exceptions. See McCormack, supra, note 15 §290.

31. The physician profile is a summary of the characteristics of a doctor's practice derived by computer analysis of the records of all his patients. V.C. Davis V.8 (1975) 528.

32. It seems that the likelihood of success under the business records exception is slight because of the second-hand nature of information: PSRO records contain information which is abstracted from a patient's medical record. Generally, second-hand recorded data cannot be used in court where first-hand or better information is readily available ("best evidence" rule calls for use of primary evidence if it is available). The patient's medical record is, therefore, a far better source of information than a PSRO record, because it contains more first-hand information and presents a more detailed record of a patient's medical status.

33. Most courts would, of course, prohibit this sort of information on public policy or statutory grounds (state, federal) if it dealt with disciplinary matters, but there is a chance that a state court may refuse to recognize federal policy or that there is no preventive state legislation.

34. If the PSRO committee recommends a physician be sanctioned and the Secretary of HEW actually does so, such information becomes a matter of public record, and as a public document can be admitted into evidence at trial.

35. McCormack, supra, note 15, §156.

36. Id.

37. Id.

38. Gonzales v. Nork, Cal. Super. Ct. # 228-566, Sacramento Co. 1973.

39. *U. Cal. at Davis,* supra, note 31.

40. For example, a physician who is recommended for exclusion from benefits by a PSRO committee may have consistently failed to conform to norms, standards, and criteria, but the nonconformity may not have resulted in any compensable injuries to a patient.

Chapter 8

Liability and the Peer Review Organization

While PSROs and other peer review organizations cannot, strictly speaking, become liable for "malpractice," they can become involved with the courts in many other kinds of cases. This chapter will explain the legal protections available to peer review groups, outline some of the most probable sources of legal difficulty for reviewers and review organizations, and, where necessary, illustrate how the law is developing, especially in regard to due-process requirements.

In which areas are reviewers most likely to run afoul of the law? This chapter will discuss negligent review, intentionally incorrect review (abuse of process), and improper communication of review results (defamation). It is not inconceivable that the review process, dealing as it does with highly sensitive information, could be thwarted by negligence, intentionally misused because of personal enmity, or result in libel or slander, whether intentional or not.

Areas of corporate liability will also be covered here. The section on corporate liability will explain how peer review organizations become liable for many of the legal mistakes of their employees and reviewers, as well as for the organization's own actions. Hospital corporate liability, an area currently in the midst of significant change, will be reviewed next, since many of the problems experienced by hospitals may also affect peer review groups. In the last section, the question of due process, a key issue in hospital law, will be reviewed in the context of peer review procedures: review, appeals, and sanctions are all areas where the potential for organizational liability is very real.

181

EFFECT OF IMMUNITY STATUTES ON REVIEW COMMITTEES

A large number of states have passed immunity statutes which act as a protection against civil liability for individuals who are members of medical peer review committees. The state immunity laws serve to insulate nonPSRO review programs from legal action, provided that these groups exercise appropriate care and operate without malice. State laws, however, vary considerably in the scope of protection they afford to review committees. Some states, such as New Jersey, limit immunity coverage to utilization review activities only.[1] The most comprehensive statutes (Minnesota, Tennessee) protect all medical review committee members and all persons who give them information.[2]

The Tennessee statute represents perhaps the most comprehensive approach, by providing that medical review committee members "shall be immune from liability to any patient, individual, or organization for furnishing information, data, reports, records to any committee or for damages resulting from any decision, opinions, actions and proceedings rendered, entered or acted upon by such committee undertaken or performed within the scope or function of the duties of such committees, if made or taken in good faith and without malice and on the basis of facts reasonably known or reasonably believed to exist." [3] Very few states presently have legislation as broad as that enacted in Tennessee. In some jurisdictions committee members must rely solely on common-law protection.

In evaluating the scope of the state immunity statutes, we must consider whether their protections extend beyond physician reviewers to other review personnel. For example, would review coordinators be protected under state immunity statutes which mainly ensure freedom from liability for committee members? Some laws, such as New York's, afford protection to specific individuals; New York law provides that "no physician, dentist, podiatrist, or optometrist or hospital administrator ... shall be liable who serves as a member of a committee." [4] Where such wording exists, nonphysician reviewers, unless named in the list, could not be considered covered by the state's immunity law. They would have to rely on the fact that their employer would be personally (or corporately) liable for any negligent conduct on their part (vicarious liability).

In reviewing the majority of state immunity statutes, we find that in their present form they provide untested and uneven levels of protection for physician reviewers. Most lawsuits against physician reviewers or review coordinators will probably allege either negligent behavior or abuse of process, and such actions are generally not granted immunity under any state protective statute. Immunity statutes may therefore be of value not for the degree of legal protection they afford, but for the incentives they provide for encouraging physicians to serve on review panels. Such immunity clauses may, however, deter some lawsuits. More importantly, they create a favorable climate in which review activities can be conducted without fear of potential legal repercussions.

REVIEWER AND COMMITTEE MEMBER NEGLIGENCE

In discussing the issue of negligence in peer review, a question of the potential liability of medical reviewers (physicians and nurses) and peer review committee members is often raised. Reviewer liability might arise in a case where a peer review organization issues a denial of admission or continued stay and, as a consequence of the denial, the patient leaves the institution and later becomes violently ill or dies. If the incident leads to a civil suit for negligence, who is responsible? Are medical reviewers and peer review committee members liable for faulty determinations, or are they protected under law? The answer to this second question depends upon whether a PSRO or other type of review group is involved. Lawsuits stemming from a faulty review decision will probably arise at the initial stages of PSRO review and at the initial committee level determinations.

Section 1167(b)(1) of the PSRO statute seems to be adequate protection against liability in a situation where a patient was incorrectly denied admission or continued stay and suffered injury because of it, if the decision was rendered with appropriate professional care. The question, therefore, is: What would constitute a lack of due care in a PSRO review context? As far as the PSRO review committee is concerned (if the review determination reaches that level), the committee is responsible for reviewing the patients' abstracts and any records presented to it. Committee members do not have to go beyond the documentation presented by the physician adviser or attending physician, unless it is obvious that the information is so inadequate or incomplete that it cannot serve as the basis for an intelligent decision. If it can be shown, however, that a PSRO committee made a decision without appropriate medical evidence, or rendered a decision that ignored the evidence, then it is possible that the committee would be held liable.

More than a lack of due care is required for a negligence lawsuit against one or more individual committee members to be successful; there must be a measurable injury to the patient resulting directly from the committee denial. For example, in the case where a PSRO committee incorrectly denies admission certification to a patient and injury results, the injury must be directly attributable to the negligent denial in order for it to be compensable. If it can be shown that the individual would have suffered harm with or without the denial, then a negligence action based on a faulty denial would have no chance of success.

The immunity protection against civil and criminal liability (1167(b)(1)) extends not only to PSRO physician-reviewers, but also to review coordinators who are employees of the PSRO, and to nonPSRO physicians and nonemployee review coordinators in delegated hospitals who could be classified as "providing professional counseling or services" to the PSRO.

In the review process, the initial screening of the patient's chart will be done by the review coordinator, whose function is to manage the review in its routine stages. The information the review coordinator obtains about a patient, and transmits to the physician adviser, is crucial to the outcome of the PSRO review. The review coordinator who fails to transmit accurate data to the medical adviser may, therefore, if injury to the patient results, be liable for failure to exercise due care.[5] There may be rare instances when due care would require the review coordinator, because of insufficient or questionable data, to recommend that the patient be seen by a PSRO physician before a determination be made.

The review coordinator has a responsibility to insure that adequate review procedures are carried out, and that the appropriate parties are contacted before review decisions are reached. The review coordinator must work in conjunction with the physician adviser and the attending physician, because the coordinator does not have the authority to make review determinations: this is the responsibility of the physician adviser. The coordinator, however, may, if the PSRO physician was negligent in not carefully reviewing the case in such a situation, be named as a party to a lawsuit where a patient sustained injury because of the denial.

The coordinator's misuse of criteria would only lead to the admission or continued stay being classified questionable and referred to the PSRO adviser for further determination. A review coordinator is more likely to be held liable for failure to follow specified review procedures than for failure to apply PSRO criteria in a given case. The coordinator uses criteria as a guide to screen each reviewed admission and can exercise some flexibility in applying those criteria. The misuse of criteria would only be meaningful in a negligence context if it resulted in an improper denial, in which case liability would fall on the PSRO adviser or committee, not the review coordinator.

The responsibility of the PSRO physician adviser as the PSRO agent is greater than that of the review coordinator. As an individual who has

statutory authority to make final PSRO determinations (if they are un-
challenged), the adviser may be exposed to a higher risk of liability.
When the review coordinator identifies a questionable admission (or the
physician adviser feels, based on his screening of a chart, that an admission is questionable), it is up to the adviser to review the merits of the
admission and to reach a final determination.

Basically, both the review coordinator and the physician adviser are
required to evaluate data's accuracy and make reasonable medical judgments based upon patients' charts, attending and specialty consultation, and the criteria established by the PSRO. In order to exercise due
care, the physician adviser must review the appropriate data (e.g., progress notes, nurses' notes). If it is apparent that the data presented for
review is inadequate, or is in such form that it cannot be interpreted by
the physician adviser, additional information must be obtained. The
physician adviser who has problems approving a given admission should
contact the attending physician for a clarification of the record, or for
additional information about the reasons for the patient's hospitalization. A failure to consult with the attending physician may, if denial results in injury, constitute a violation of what in the review situation
could be considered due care. When the attending physician and PSRO
adviser cannot agree, it may be necessary to obtain a second opinion,
particularly in the case of certain specialties. Failure to obtain a necessary second opinion may be a basis, in some cases, for a finding of negligence. Instances could arise where the PSRO physician adviser (or
supervisor) may wish, before a determination is reached, to have a consultant examine the patient in question. But examination of the patient
by the PSRO will probably be quite rare and would ordinarily not occur
without the attending physician's permission; and, for purposes of exercising due care, it should not be necessary.

Adequate record keeping is a basic concern for all peer review
programs. In the case of a review denial, it is especially important that
sufficient documentation be provided so that the reasons can be clearly
identified by anyone examining the record. Too often the documentation of inhospital U.R. review committees tends to be insufficient, and
many of these committees would be hard pressed to demonstrate on the
basis of their records that they exercised due care in their review function. One may argue that review in its initial phases should be conducted in an informal manner, but this fact does not obviate the legal
need for precise record keeping.

Failure to keep accurate records on the part of the peer review organization would not in and of itself create liability, but it would certainly
hinder any organization involved in an adversary proceeding from

demonstrating that it exercised due care in a given instance. While identifiable PSRO records may be protected from subpoena, that policy should not be relied on to negate the responsibility to keep accurate records, especially in the case of a denial or sanction. If a contested denial reaches a federal court, the involved patient's peer review record may be brought into the proceeding as essential, or, at the least, material, evidence to be reviewed by the judge or jury. Poor documentation would hardly aid the PSRO in demonstrating the exercise of due care.[6] During the internal PSRO appeals process, a need, therefore, exists for complete and accurate documentation, because oral testimony alone will prove that the case in question was properly reviewed.

In the event a patient is improperly denied admission to or continued stay in a hospital, does the patient have legal recourse if he or she fails to appeal that determination through the PSRO system? While a patient has the right to seek "internal" review of a PSRO denial, that right does not preclude a negligence lawsuit against individual reviewers and/or the PSRO committee. Appeal through the PSRO system is necessary if the patient wishes to obtain an overruling of a PSRO denial and receive retrospective reimbursement, but the patient may have other concerns besides the money involved. In classifying a determination as incorrect, the PSRO appellate process does not identify fault in the same sense a negligence action would. The fact that an appeals panel uncovers a faulty review decision does not mean that that particular decision was rendered negligently. If a patient wishes to assign blame, or recover damages, a lawsuit would be the best recourse. The reviewer or committee member who is sued for negligence could not expect to rely on the fact that a patient did not appeal a denial in the PSRO system as a defense.[7]

ABUSE OF PROCESS

Whether or not there has been a violation of due care (i.e., negligent conduct), liability can arise in the review situation whenever it can be demonstrated that the reviewer or review committee acted with malice.[8] Malice, in and of itself, is not a legal cause of action, but rather an element of a number of civil and criminal actions. While malicious behavior may be present in defamation, or in a violation of due process, in most instances a purposeful intent to harm on the part of a committee reviewer could be construed as an "abuse of process."

This tort, abuse of process, is defined as "the employment of a process in a manner not contemplated by law or to obtain an object which such a process is not intended by law to effect." [9] It should be noted that in order for a lawsuit for abuse of process to succeed, there must be a measurable harm or injury to the plaintiff. The law infers the existence of malice from the willfull or intentional conduct of the defendant.

Abuses of review procedures would be more likely to occur at the peer review committee level than in the initial stages of review. Because review coordinators do not make final determinations, it would be difficult for most coordinators to be liable for abuse of process, although there is always the possibility that one could purposefully thwart the system in such a way as to harm an individual physician. [10] The likelihood of a physician adviser misusing the system to harm a colleague would depend upon the review group's organizational structure, and on the influence of the individual reviewer. At the PSRO committee level, an influential physician, or group of physicians, could conceivably manipulate the process against a given individual more successfully than at lower levels of review. The likelihood of a PSRO reviewer or committee member thwarting the process for malicious reasons is remote, but if it does occur the PSRO law does not afford immunity protection.

DEFAMATION

The PSRO's responsibility to recommend to HEW, where necessary, the sanctioning of a physician (§1160(b)(1)) could conceivably lead to a situation in which an individual is maliciously and falsely singled out for disciplinary action. The perversion of the review process in this manner can give rise to a lawsuit for defamation.

The Law of Defamation

Defamation is defined as "that which tends to injure reputation in the popular sense, to diminish the esteem, respect, good will or confidence in which the plaintiff is held or to excite adverse derogatory or unpleasant feelings or opinions against him. [11] Defamation is a term which includes both libel and slander, the former being actionable conduct stemming from written or printed words, the latter, actionable conduct stemming from spoken words or gestures.

To win a lawsuit for defamation, the plaintiff must prove the following: that the communication is defamatory, published (shown or told to someone else), applicable to the plaintiff, understood as applying to the plaintiff, and causes measurable harm. [12] It is important to remember that liability may exist even where the defendant is ignorant of the defamatory nature of his statement. In other words, the defamer's state of mind is unimportant: in the common law, if a statement *is* defamatory (i.e., understood or understandable by others as libel or slander), it makes no difference that the person making the untrue statement did not intend it to be defamatory. State of mind (malice, reasonable belief, etc.) does become important, however, where the defamation occurs in a situation in which the defamer has a "qualified privilege" to make statements on certain subjects.

Under the law, both judicial and statutory, there are instances when legal protection is afforded to all statements, including those that are defamatory. These include statements made in certain forums such as court or a legislative hearing. Statements made in such places are deemed to be "absolutely privileged".[13] However, most of the privileges that can be raised as defenses against liability for defamation are "conditional" or "qualified." This means that the law recognizes that the statements were made in pursuance of some duty (i.e., a legal or moral responsibility) or in connection with some matter in which the speaker had an interest. They therefore should not render the speaker or writer open to suit unless the statements were malicious as well as untrue.[14] Some qualified privileges have been created by the courts; some arise from statutes.

Common Law Defenses

The chances that a court would apply the doctrine of absolute privilege to the peer review situation, on the argument that such process constitutes a quasi-judicial review, are remote at best. It is probably inaccurate to label peer review committee meetings as quasi-judicial in nature: few or none of the protections inherent in judicial proceedings are available to the reviewed physician/practitioner.

The claim of conditional privilege in the medical review situation would best fit into the classification of "common interest," a doctrine that covers communications between and among individuals who share a mutual interest wherever the communication is of a kind reasonably calculated to protect or further that interest.[15] At one time the defense of a "privilege based on a common interest" was deemed to be limited to pecuniary matters, but the doctrine has been expanded to include the interests of professional groups. It should be noted that, according to legal authority, "the conditional privilege is lost if the defamation goes beyond the group interest or if publication is made to persons who have no reason to receive the information.[16]

In other words, in a medical review situation, a review coordinator who inadvertently defames a physician by passing false review information to a physician adviser would be protected because the exchanging of information about care is within the common interest of both parties in the process. If it can be shown that the review coordinator acted with malice in passing the defamatory misinformation to the physician adviser, and the latter party accepted it as true, this would suffice to destroy the conditional privilege. As the court held in *Shapiro v. HIP*, "When a defendant's statements are presumptively privileged, the rule is that, in order to render them actionable it is incumbent on the plaintiff to prove that they were false and that the defendant was actuated by express malice or actual ill will." [17] Similarly, if it can be demonstrated that the review coordinator or physician adviser has disseminated defamatory misinformation outside the review organization, the privilege would be broken. For example, if a physician adviser, even if well-intentioned, gives defamatory matter concerning a staff member to the local medical society this would be passing data to a group not directly involved in the review process. [18]

In short, at all levels of peer review the qualified privilege can be invoked to protect those involved from potential liability for defamation, provided the communication is not intentionally malicious. Statements and reports issued by a PSRO during a sanctioning proceeding are protected by a qualified privilege, unless those reports are leaked to improper sources or are clearly falsified. In a case where defamation is found and no privilege exists, both the individual who defamed the plaintiff and PSRO itself would be held liable.

It cannot be overemphasized that PSROs must be aware that the information with which they deal is sensitive, and that confidentiality of personally identifiable data must be upheld, not only to protect individual privacy, but to protect the PSRO from liability. It should be a basic tenet of the review organization that care must be taken by PSRO personnel (reviewers and committee members) not to discuss privileged matter outside the organization, whether or not a sanction is being considered. It is entirely conceivable that a careless disclosure of sensitive information by a review committee member to an uninvolved colleague could be the initial event that triggers a defamation suit.

There is surprisingly little precedent on the question of privilege to defame in the course of medical practice. Most of the defamation cases dealing with physicians concern the question of whether defamatory communications made by a physician about a patient fall within the protection of a qualified privilege. However, the New York Court of Appeals' case of *Shapiro v. Health Insurance Plan of Greater New York*,[19] a suit for defamation by a surgeon against a health insurance company, represents a close parallel to a defamation suit against a medical review group. The court in the Shapiro case ruled that the statements, oral and written, issued by a health insurer were covered by qualified privilege; therefore, to overcome that privilege there had to be a showing of malice.

Said the court: "Defendants (HIP) had a duty and a right to investigate and communicate the results of their investigation to other similarly interested persons. Those communications were privileged unless made because of malice. It was for the plaintiff to show that he had facts available to prove malice. Suspicion, surmise, and accusation are not enough. The existence of earlier disputes between the parties is not evidence of malice." The New York Court stated that malice is "consistent with the desire to injure the plaintiff . . . by actual malice is meant personal spite or ill will or culpable recklessness or negligence." [20] If the logic of Shapiro and similar cases is persuasive in the peer review situation, it will be necessary to show that a reviewer or committee acted out of the scope of its authority or interest, or was motivated by malice in fact.[21]

Statutory Defenses

The second line of defense for defamation suits against a peer review organization or hospital can be based on state immunity statutes, which, as previously noted, provide inconsistent levels of protection. PSROs have available to them the additional special immunities of §§1167(a) and (b) of the Social Security Act. Section 1167(a) is designed to protect individuals who give information to the PSRO:

> No person providing information to any Professional Standards Review Organization shall be held, by reason for having provided such information, to have violated any criminal law or to be civilly liable unless (1) such information is unrelated to the performance of the duties and functions of such organization or (2) such information is false and the person providing such information knew, or had reason to believe, that such information was false.

In other words, the qualified privilege created by §1167(a), although it is available to individuals both inside and outside the PSRO, is limited to materials demanded by the review process, and applies only when the falsification (and therefore defamation) is inadvertent.

Section 1167(b) does not provide protection against intentional defamation, because the section's immunities are available only as long as due care is exercised and there is an absence of malice. Unintentional defamation is again protected, and the protection extends to anyone who is "a member or employee" of any PSRO, or who "furnishes professional counsel or services" to it.[22] Although §1167(b) does not refer specifically to the giving or receiving of information pursuant to the review process, it does cover "the performance . . . of any duty, function, or activity authorized or required" [23] by the PSRO law, which would presumably include transmitting information; so that, at least as regards legal protection against suits for defamation, subsections (a) and (b) of §1167 do not conflict.

It should be obvious that §§1167(a) and (b) closely parallel the common law of conditional privilege. Thus the legal effect of the statute is to create a conditional privilege for the communication of information, including defamatory information, which does not require a court to first find, or invent, a basis for that conditional privilege.[24]

We should also note that §1167's partial protection of defamation is somewhat mitigated by §1166, which, by authorizing fines and/or imprisonment for unauthorized disclosures, should reduce the potential scope of publication.

CORPORATE LIABILITY OF PEER REVIEW ORGANIZATIONS

General Principles

The question of the liabilities of the reviewers and committee members leads to the much broader issue of the potential liability of the peer review organization itself. For example, is the PSRO as a whole liable for the torts of its employees? Certainly the PSRO, as a corporate entity, does have legal responsibilities for which it can be held accountable under state and federal law, but there are special limits to PSROs' liability.

The nature and extent of corporate liability varies with the type of organization. For example, an institutional peer review committee is not liable in and of itself, although of course its members may be individually liable; rather, responsibility ultimately rests with the parent institution.

Corporate negligence has been defined as "the failure of those entrusted with the task of providing the accommodations and facilities necessary to carry out the purposes of the corporation to follow in a given situation the established standard of conduct to which the corporation should conform."[25] A corporation as an entity is liable for the failure by its directors, officers, and/or employees to carry out legally required duties and functions.

Under the doctrine of *respondeat superior*, an employer is legally responsible for the wrongdoings of an employee. That is not to say, however, that those individuals acting on behalf of the PSRO are not personally liable for tortious conduct committed in the course of employment. For example, a medical director who defames a local physician in an official PSRO report has created a potential liability for both himself and the organization.

PSROs' Organizational Liability

In considering the liability of peer review organizations, we are concerned with those actions on the part of the board of directors, medical and executive directors, officers and employees in their capacity as corporate agents that may lead to organizational liability. In the case of the PSRO, it is not difficult to ascertain the organization's corporate responsibilities on the basis of specified duties delineated in the federal law and in each organization's articles of incorporation and by-laws.

PSRO corporate liability problems presently would include suits for defamation; improper release of information (including suits to enjoin information release as well as suits for damages); faulty review; improper development of review guidelines; failure to sanction; failure to delegate; failure to grant due process rights, etc. HEW has only recently begun to come to grips with the possibility of PSRO liability. Its first affirmative actions have been to: (1) aid PSROs in obtaining insurance coverage and (2) promise to provide legal assistance to PSROs that are sued.[26] The federal government has taken the position that it does not have the legislative authority to indemnify PSROs or individuals within PSROs for damages awarded against them.[27]

While individuals working for PSROs or similar organizations may be afforded some protection by virtue of state and, in the case of PSROs, federal immunity statutes, most immunity statutes are directed toward protecting only individuals; it is highly improbable that PSROs would qualify for status as individual personages. The PSRO statute's §1167(b)(1) clearly refers only to individual persons and not to corporations.

Can an individual's legal immunity from liability be transferred to the PSRO or other review group under state law? If members of a PSRO board of directors are named as defendants in a lawsuit, and the immunity section prevents the directors from liability, can §1167 be used to protect the PSRO as a corporate entity? Under both the law of agency and the law of tort, immunities from liability cannot be transferred from the agent to the principal (i.e., from the employee to the employer).

Says the American Law Institute, "Where the principal directs an agent to act or the agent acts in a scope of employment, the fact that the agent has an immunity from liability does not bar a civil action against the principal."[28] Similarly, the American Law Institute Restatement of Torts states that "where two persons would otherwise be liable for a harm, one of them is not relieved from liability by the fact that the other has absolute privilege to act or an immunity from liability to the person harmed."[29] Thus, the PSRO or review organization operating under a similar immunity statute cannot claim freedom from immunity by virtue of §1167(b)(1) or similar language in a state statute, but may be held liable, as a corporation, for occurrences for which its employees are protected.

Individuals in the PSRO who are involved in corporate decision-making activities, such as the executive or the medical director, will be protected from liability, provided they exercise due care, by virtue of the PSRO immunity statute. The question may also arise as to whether the PSRO board of directors, who are engaged in overseeing the PSRO's business and property interests, are protected by the immunity statute in carrying out their responsibilities. The answer appears to be "yes." The statutory language does not exclude them, and the Senate Finance Committee Report, in dealing with §1167, states that, "the intention of the provision . . . is to remove any inhibition to proper exercise of PSRO functions," and that coverage is not limited to review activities.[30]

While the PSRO immunity section may protect the PSRO's board of directors, it is doubtful whether state immunity laws are specifically directed toward medical review committee activities; they do not extend to the business operations of a review entity. A board of directors of a review organization that came under the jurisdiction of state law would have to rely on either the statutory or common law of that jurisdiction for possible protection. A PSRO, as a nonprofit state-incorporated entity, will fall under a given state's corporate laws, and it will often be the responsibility of a state court to recognize that the federal immunity provision has precedence over state law in questions of individual liability for corporate error.

HOSPITAL CORPORATE LIABILITY

In assessing the PSRO's potential liability, it is helpful to review some of the changes that have occurred in the common law of hospital corporate liability. The duties of the hospital toward the patient, the medical staff, and the community at large have all been broadened by developments in legislative and common law. The focus of this chapter is on only one area of developing hospital corporate responsibility: the hospital's growing responsibility to ensure adequate-quality medical care in the institution.

In 1965 an Illinois appellate court, in *Darling v. Charlestown Community Memorial Hospital,* ruled that it was the responsibility of the hospital to monitor and ensure adequate health care in the institution.[31] The Supreme Court of Nevada, in *Moore v. Board of Trustees of Carson Tahoe Hospital,* stated that "the purpose of the Community Hospital is to provide patient care of the highest possible quality."[32] To implement this duty of providing competent medical care to the patients, it is the institution's responsibility to create a workable system whereby the medical staff continually reviews and evaluates the quality of care. In *Gonzales v. Nork,*[33] a California trial court required that some type of peer review be employed within the hospital to ensure that the patients received quality care. A New Jersey court went so far as to rule that the duty to review the performance of a physician in the institution rested not only on the hospital as a corporation, but also on the hospital's entire medical staff.[34]

Those courts that have required some type of internal medical review did not develop such a doctrine independently, but based it on review programs emanating from professional groups, such as the JCAH, and later from legislation. In the words of an article in the *California Western Law Review:*[35] "The courts ... in response to standards of hospital accreditation developed by professionals in medicine and in hospital administration, recognized that the hospital is openly responsible to the public for both the cost and the quality of health care." The Arizona Court of Appeals, in *Purcell v. Zimbelman,*[36] in ruling that the hospital was responsible for its own quality of care, based the decision upon hospital accreditation standards. While only a small minority of jurisdictions have expanded hospital responsibility to the extent of these court decisions, there is an identifiable trend toward increasing the hospital's responsibility for medical care.

With the continued expansion of medical peer review programs, it is reasonable to expect that courts will look to these programs in assessing the responsibilities of health care institutions. Hospitals in all jurisdictions must develop adequate peer review systems, not only to adhere to legislative requirements, but to comply with the expanding common-law duty. The adoption of a requirement that hospitals monitor the quality of their medical care should act as an incentive to strengthen and develop peer review programs.

The effect of hospital corporate law on the liability of peer review organizations is not easy to assess. It would seem at present to create a legal analogy, although not a precedent, for expanding the scope of responsibilities of medical review organizations of any type. However, there is one area of activity in hospital corporate law that may have direct ramifications on the present operation of PSROs: The area of physician due process rights inhering in a review situation.

DUE PROCESS AND PEER REVIEW

During Initial Review

While the hospitals' common-law and statutory duties to monitor the quality of health care have expanded, there has been a growing awareness that the institution, in carrying out its function of review, must afford physicians the right to be protected from arbitrary or unreasonable decision-making. Physicians involved in disciplinary (e.g., reduction-of-privilege) hearings must be granted procedural due process rights.[37, 38]

As far as medical case law is concerned, the courts have increasingly tended to refrain from becoming involved in internal hospital procedural matters, provided the hospital has established a mechanism for ensuring that physicians' rights are upheld in any hearing process. Where a clear violation of due process is present (i.e., a failure to use the hearing procedure specified or a fundamental unfairness in the process), courts will find the hospital liable for denying the rights of staff members. For example, in *Visalli v. Mary's Help Hospital*,[39] a California court awarded the plaintiff surgeon $200,000 on the ground that the hospital peer review committee violated his due process rights. The Visalli court felt that the review committee had unjustifiably placed the plaintifi on review for an overly extended period of time when there was no empirical evidence of misconduct or "poor practice," and that this delay had resulted in serious harm to the plantiff.

Appeals

Clearly, a peer review organization must be concerned with the due process rights of physicians on review, as failure to grant such rights may lead to liability (as is true in a hospital review situation). Appeals and sanctions are especially sensitive areas in which PSROs are going to have to concern themselves with ensuring that procedural guarantees of fairness are enforced.

The PSRO appeals system, as it is presently constituted, involves a multileveled structure in which an aggrieved party can conceivably pursue his claim before five different administrative hearing panels, during a time period extending well beyond one year. Review beyond reconsideration was originally to be limited to patients, but the policy was changed so that physicians and institutions were allowed to enter appeals: these later groups are more likely to pursue claims because of financial incentives.[40]

There are several problems with pursuing a PSRO appeal in a federal court, the first of which is the amount of time required to reach this level of relief. In order to appeal in federal court a decision rendered in an administrative process, all the procedures in that process must first have been exhausted. When the plaintiff moves from an administrative forum into a legal one, the court will generally not review factual determinations made by the administrative panel; and it is probable that most PSRO claims will involve factual rather than legal issues. Ordinarily, the federal court's only responsibility is to determine whether errors of law have occurred in the administrative hearing process, and the court will review facts only to the extent necessary to make such a determination.

Nevertheless, plaintiffs can occasionally obtain broader review. An individual can possibly challenge the regulations governing appeals as being arbitrary and capricious, and in this way force the court to examine the factual issues in greater detail. But an administrative panel lacks the authority to declare the regulatory structure under which it operates illegal. Also, the plaintiff could ask for injunctive relief, claiming that the administrative panel failed to follow its own regulations, and thus, if successful, return the case to the administrative process for a rehearing.

It is essential that as the PSRO appeal is carried out, the individual's fundamental (due process) rights are adhered to. Generally, if PSROs establish a well-defined system of review that affords all of the parties involved equitable recourse, courts will not readily invalidate the organizations' internal due process. Failure on the part of the PSRO to establish a well-defined process for reconsiderations, or error in implementing review procedures, could lead to organizational liability. For example, failure to notify a patient of his right to appeal and that the PSRO will assist him, or use of interested parties as medical reviewers, could constitute potential grounds for a due process violation.

A fundamental issue in assessing the relationship of due process to the PSRO appeals system is whether the system as a whole is fundamentally fair. A strong argument could be made that in the case of a patient claimant, a review process that could extend for a lengthy time period and involve several hearings, may, in fact, impose a severe personal hardship in loss of both time and income. A person who is medically incapacitated may lack the ability to deal adequately with this rather complex administrative review structure. While the PSRO may provide some assistance to the patient claimant in preparing the appeal, that assistance, coming from an interested party, may not be without bias. The appeals system, as it is now developing, poses a potential hardship to the average patient and may deny fundamental rights.

To avoid due process difficulties inherent in the present structure, the PSRO's appellate review should be limited to three administrative stages, with only one stage involving outside review; the time span for the review process should be shortened; and any patient wishing to appeal should have his case handled by an appellate representative who has had no contact with the PSRO. The PSRO should both provide the patient with formal notice of the right to appeal, and require the patient to sign a form attesting that he understood the notice of denial and the right to appeal.

Sanctions

The PSRO has a statutory duty to uncover and report deviant practitioners to either the state PSR Council or to the Secretary of HEW directly.[41] The failure of the PSRO to carry out its sanctioning responsibility could lead to organizational liability. The ability of the PSRO and other peer review groups to sanction or discipline is crucial to the organization's ultimate effectiveness. While review bodies are not designed as disciplinary entities, if they are working adequately they will probably uncover problem areas where, in some instances, extreme measures will be needed to effect changes in medical practice.

Successful handling of medical problem areas will present a delicate task for the PSRO; ideally, this can be done in an informal manner, as recommended in HEW's draft guidelines.[42] When the PSRO must take disciplinary measures, it must be very cautious, proceeding along a clearly defined course of action which affords the deviant physician his legal rights. A practitioner who is denied the ability to be paid under Title XVIII and XIX programs will, no doubt, attempt to protect his interests. He may not hesitate to sue the PSRO, particularly if the practitioner feels that he was dealt with unfairly or in an arbitrary manner.[43]

That HEW rather than the PSRO has the power to punish, discipline, and sanction may account for the lack of any formal hearing, appeal, or appeal requirement at the PSRO or State PSR Council level. The only formal hearing and appeal that a party to a sanction action can raise in the administrative system is at the Secretarial level.[44] PSRO procedures adopted in disciplinary investigations, while generally informal, must be carefully defined and followed if the PSRO is to survive challenges on the grounds of failure to grant due process rights. As is the case in the appeals system, a sanctioned physician or institution has the right to seek redress in federal court, and it is not unthinkable that the claimant in a court action will raise the issue of failure to grant due process of law at the PSRO level.

NOTES

1. N.J. Stat. Ann. Sec. 2A:84A-22.8-22.9 (Supp. 1974).

2. Minn.—Second Regular Session Laws, 1974, Ch. 295; Tenn. Code Ann. Vol. IIA. Sec. 63-623 (Supp. 1974).

3. Id. at Tennessee 63.623.

4. N.Y. Educ. Law Sec. 6527 (3) (McKinney Supp. 1973).

5. Furthermore, the review coordinator must make sure the documentation supplied by the admitting physician is adequate; if it is not, the coordinator should check with the physician adviser or a PSRO consultant.

6. Similarly, in a case in which a physician sues a PSRO for improperly recommending sanctions (perhaps on a defamation theory), the record of the PSRO sanctioning proceeding may be required for use in court.

7. Bureau of Quality Assurance, *PSRO Manual*, Chapt. 19.

8. A malicious act involves the willful disregard of the rights of another to encompass either some unlawful end or a lawful end by unlawful means. It is important to recognize that malice is to be distinguished from negligent behavior in that malice requires a purposeful intention, whereas the essence of negligence is inadvertence (absence of intent to injure). Malice in law can be derived inferentially from the surrounding circumstances.

9. "Abuse of Process" 41 Am. Jur.2d.(1968): "Elements essential to sustain the action are: (1) That the defendant made an illegal, improper, or perverted use of the process, a use neither warranted nor authorized by the process; (2) that the defendant had an ulterior motive or purpose in exercising such illegal, perverted or improper use of process; and (3) that damage resulted to the plaintiff from the irregularity."

10. The physician on review always has the option to go directly to the PSRO to complain or appeal if he/she feels harassment.

11. Prosser, *Law of Torts* (St. Paul: West), p. 739.

12. Addis, W.T., *Torts* (Philadelphia: Levin-Sarner-Brown, 1974), p. 56.

13. Prosser, §114 p. 777.

14. Id, §115.

15. Id.

16. Id. at 792.

17. Shapiro v. HIP 197 N.Y.S.2d 509 (1959).

18. There may be instances where the physician advisor would feel information that turns out to be defamatory should be passed on to the hospital's administration or department

chairman: this may be possible under hospital by-laws or the general group interest theory.

19. Shapiro, supra, note 17.

20. Id.

21. The legal doctrine of malice in law won't hold up here because more than a showing of presumed malice is required before the qualified privilege can be negated.

22. P.L. 92-603 §1167(b)(1).

23. Id.

24. Prosser, §115.

25. Bader v. United Orthodox Synagogue, 172 A.2d 192, 194 (1961 Comm.).

26. *Internal Medicine News,* Nov. 15, 1975.

27. At this early stage in the PSRO program, few lawsuits have occurred. One PSRO has been sued for failure to delegate a small hospital (Frank R. Howard Memorial Hospital v. Redwood Coast PSRO). The hospital that sued the Redwood Coast PSRO based its case on the fact that the PSRO denial did not rest on any legitimate grounds. *The PSRO Manual* (Chapter 7) and Transmittal Letter No. 11 do not discuss the size of the hospital as a criterion for denial of delegated status, although, in fact, it may be a legitimate consideration. This suit was settled out of court by the PSRO, resulting in the organization's granting delegated status to the plaintiff hospital.

If the Federal Tort Claims Act is applied to PSROs, it will then become the responsibility of the PSRO to indemnify any individuals who are injured as a result of the negligence of a PSRO employee.

28. American Law Institute, *Restatement of the Law of Agency 2d* (St. Paul. West, 1958), §217.

29. American Law Institute, *Restatement of the Law of Torts* (St. Paul: American Law Institute Publishers, 1939), §880.

30. *Report of the Senate Finance Committee* No. 92, p. 1230.

31. Darling v. Charlestown Community Memorial Hospital, 33 I11.2d 326. (1965).

32. Moore v. Board of Trustees of Carson Tahoe Hospital, 495 P.2d 605 (1972).

33. Gonzales v. Nork, Cal. Super. Ct. #228-566, Sacramento Co., 1973.

34. Corletto v. South Shore Memorial Hospital 138 N.J. Super.302, 350 A.2d 534 (1976).

35. Arthur Southwick, "The Hospital as an Institution—Expanding Responsibilities Change Its Relationship with the Staff Physician," *California Western Law Review* 9 (1973), p. 429.

36. Purcell v. Zimbelman 18 Ariz. App. 75, 500 P.2d 335 (1972).

37. Procedural due process in the medical review context has been defined by the Supreme Court of Hawaii in Silver v. Castle Memorial Hospital to include: (1) notice of the availability of a hearing; (2) adequate notice of the time and place of the hearing; (3) specific statement of charges or issues to be discussed; (4) opportunity to present and cross examine witnesses; (5) representation by counsel (if other party is so represented); (6) decision firmly based on facts presented; and (7) communication of the decision in writing. (See 497 P. 2d 573 (1972).)

38. The distinction between public and private hospitals for purposes of providing due process guarantees (state action concept) is no longer applicable in all jurisdictions. Many courts treat private hospitals as quasi-public because of the amount of funding they receive from government sources; thus, private institutions are required to conform to the same standards of procedural fairness as public hospitals. Moreover, the Joint Commis-

sion on the Accreditation of Hospitals *Guidelines for the Formulation of Medical Staff By-Laws, Rules and Regulations* carefully provide for due process of law with respect to medical staff appointments and privileges.

39. Visalli v. Mary's Help Hospital, Superior Ct. Calif., San Mateo County, No. 151, 707 (1975).

40. *PSRO Manual*, Chapt. 19. After a denial has been made, the initial appeal can be raised by the attending physician, the patient, or the institution within three days. The initial appeal hearing and the reconsideration hearing will be similar: The reviewers involved must have no prior connection with the case, and must be drawn from the appropriate specialty. The parties will have access to necessary records (even if the data therein is confidential), have the right to present oral and written evidence at a hearing, and be represented by another party if they so desire. In the event of an adverse decision, all of the parties plus the appropriate fiscal intermediary or state agency will be notified of the decision and reasons for it; payment will cease within 24 hours after the determination. The parties must also be informed of their continued rights of appeal, and patients who need assistance will be aided by the PSRO in preparing their claim.

As the process moves outside of the individual PSRO, it goes to a state PSR Council hearing (if such a council exists in a state) where the case record will be reviewed to determine this stage. Beyond the state PSR Council, one can carry the claim to the Secretary of HEW, where the case will be handled by the Bureau of Hearings and Appeals within the Social Security Administration. The initial appeal at the Secretary's level will be handled by a hearing judge, who will conduct an administrative hearing in which the patient may present oral and written evidence. If the patient receives an adverse determination from the hearing examiner, he may bring the case before the Appeals Council in the Social Security Administration system, which body will review the record to determine if reversible error is present. The second level of appeal within SSA is the last stage in the administrative review; once completed, the claimant may seek relief in a federal court, provided the amount in controversy exceeds one thousand dollars. (See Chapter 19, *PSRO Manual.*) See also BQA "Draft Proposed Statewide Council Appeals Procedure," Dec. 1976.

41. DHEW, *PSRO Manual*, CH.20, "Sanctions" (Washington: BQA, 1976).

42. Id.

43. In order for the PSRO to recommend sanctions, there must be strong evidence of the existence of one or more violations of PSRO guidelines, reasonable notice and opportunity for discussion with the party recommended for sanction, and a determination that the party involved was unwilling to fulfill PSRO obligations. It is especially important that the party involved be made fully aware of the inappropriate nature of his behavior, and is given a reasonable opportunity (time period) to take corrective action. Failure by the PSRO to inform an individual in an adequate fashion (in writing) that the PSRO is considering recommending sanctions would be grounds to establish an argument for violation of due process.

44. That is not to say that HEW may not require PSROs and state PSR Councils, at some future time, to hold formal hearings before recommending sanctions.

Chapter 9

Conclusion

To members of the medical professions, peer review can be an opportunity and a threat. If those who see it as a threat go to the courts for legal protection, they may find that the law not only decreases the threat but also limits the opportunities. PSROs, being a comparatively new type of peer review organization, may be particularly vulnerable to legal second-guessing.

In Chapter 1 we described medical peer review functionally: how does it work? what is it for? In this chapter, we will try to complete its legal description: what can it do? where can it go from here?

REVIEW PROGRAMS AND THE LAW TODAY

To repeat: there has been very little litigation involving peer review programs. The PSRO program has engendered few suits, of which the first three involved hospital delegation, area designation, and the constitutionality and legality of the PSRO statute. The first was settled; the second was won at trial but then mooted by a change in the statute, and never got to the appellate court; and the third, while heard by an appellate court and reported, conflicts to some extent with another decision in the same circuit court.[1] As a result, there is as yet very little precedent to limit PSRO operations in any way.

Private-sector peer review programs—primarily those which are hospital-based—have been in court somewhat more frequently, with the result that a lawyer who counsels any peer review group, whether public or private, can point to legal precedent (at least in some jurisdictions) in favor of the following positions:

- The review group's hearings and appeals procedures should follow at least minimal due process standards, probably including impar-

201

tial and unbiased hearing/appeal panels, reasonably speedy procedures, and adequate notification to any disciplined or suspect physician (which probably means a written statement of what action is being taken or contemplated, why, and what the physician's next step(s) should be if he wishes to contest the decision). The review group would also be in a safer legal position if its procedures were written and distributed to all potential participants *before* the procedures were needed, rather than developed on an *ad hoc* basis after a conflict has arisen. Although in most cases advance notification of the group's intended procedures is not absolutely necessary —merely highly desirable—the group that decides to simplify its organizational effort by relying on *ad hoc* procedures "if and when" may be saving time at the expense of drastically increased litigation costs in the future.

- The group and its employees and agents (reviewers) should avoid defaming the people and institutions it reviews, and in general should release review results, favorable or not, only to those who have a right to be told those results. Of course, if the courts determine that the public has that right, the group need not worry as much about the law, although its relationship with the hospitals and physicians in its area may suffer. While it should be obvious that a review group should not try to gain access to any patients' records to which it is not entitled, some may be tempted, particularly where medical audit (an MCE) is being performed, to look at the charts of otherwise nonreviewable patients in order to increase the size of the review sample. The law of privacy is in flux, and it is not clear that a hospital can release a patient's record to an outside review group without the patient's express permission, unless, as is the case for PSROs, a federal or state law gives the review group the right to proceed without that permission.

- The group must avoid negligence: the reviewer or review committee has a legal duty to give each case before it enough time and attention so that it can make a fair decision based on the facts in the chart or (if procedures allow it) otherwise made available to the committee. If one of the review group's coordinators or reviewers is intentionally misusing his or her position to harm a physician, or even an entire institution, that person should be replaced. The organization should establish adequate accounting procedures: misuse of federal or private funds can be a criminal offense for which the review group's directors (trustees) can be individually liable.

For PSROs the list is, naturally, more complex, because PSROs are bound by detailed "agreements" and regulations, and their ability to be in violation of a law, or in breach of a contract, is therefore increased. While the discussion in Chapter 2 was designed to make the PSRO statute more comprehensible, it should not be mistaken for legal advice. To solve legal problems or choose between operational alternatives, the advice of a lawyer who is familiar with the facts must be considered as necessary for PSROs as for any other organization.

While it is clear that "the law" does have some current application to peer review organizations' operations, the effect of peer review on the law remains problematical. Statute law has been more responsive to the existence of peer review than has the common law. In increasing numbers of states, the legislature has responded to the existence of peer review groups by enacting statutes which prohibit the use of many types of review-related documents in trials, restricting the admissibility of potentially valid and valuable evidence in order to permit reviewers to perform their jobs without fear of unnecessary involvement in litigation. In some jurisdictions, the courts have created a similar restriction without waiting for a statute to be enacted.

In general, however, it is too early to assess courts' responses to peer review. Part of the reason for this is that litigants are usually reluctant to break new ground: it is easier—and safer—to rely on precedent than to create it. Except in the handful of cases where the review program itself is the subject of litigation, peer review is rarely mentioned. We know of no cases in which either the plaintiff or defendant has attempted to introduce peer review criteria into evidence to establish medical standards. The use of expert witnesses apparently remains necessary at this time for the in-court definition of community and specialty standards of practice. As for peer review profiles or other review-generated evidence of individual medical behavior, one finds a comparative handful of malpractice cases in which such data is discussed, much less relied upon, and many of those are cases in which a hospital is being sued for corporate negligence at the same time the physician is being sued for malpractice.

Peer review results are, however, at issue in an increasing number of hospital medical staff cases, probably because an increasing number of hospitals are attempting to use peer review to rid themselves of incompetent or marginal medical staff members before those staff members' activities give rise to malpractice suits. It is not clear whether or not licensure boards are admitting peer review profiles into evidence in disciplinary proceedings, although some peer review groups have indicated their desire to offer such evidence to their respective licensure authorities after their review has uncovered clear evidence of fraud or quackery.

THE FUTURE OF PEER REVIEW LAW

As this brief review of the present state of peer review law should indicate, knowing where the law is—useful as that may be—is perhaps less useful than having some idea of where it will go. As we have tried to indicate throughout this book, there are a number of areas where change is possible. Examples include the law of privacy as it affects peer review groups' operations, the laws of evidence, and the laws applying federal administrative procedures to allegedly "private" groups. Knowing where change is possible, of course, is not the same thing as knowing where it is probable. In order to make any evaluation of the future of peer review law, however, one must necessarily make some predictions about where peer review itself is likely to cause legal trouble.

PSROs

The first question to ask in discussing changes in PSRO law is: Will the PSRO program survive? The answer is to a great extent beyond the scope of this book, depending as it does on the political and financial pressures on Congress. Senator Wallace Bennett, the PSRO law's sponsor and perhaps its strongest Congressional supporter, has retired, and the PSRO program appears to be in partial political eclipse, although this could change if Congressional attention refocuses on national health insurance or the high costs of Medicare and Medicaid. The PSRO program's political future is somewhat complicated by its lack of a constituency. Among fiscal conservatives, who might be expected to approve its cost-cutting potential, it may be viewed as too little and too late, or simply ignored as being "part of the welfare mess;" among pro-welfare liberals, it may be seen as unnecessary, too cost-conscious and insufficiently quality-conscious, or doomed to fail because of its close ties to, and dependence on, the professionals it was designed to regulate. With few to speak for it and many against it, the PSRO program may be doomed indeed.

Nevertheless, federal programs, once enacted, tend to survive, although their ultimate appearance and abilities may differ from those which the original drafters intended. It is probably safe to assume that Congress will maintain the program in some form, and, as Chapter 4 indicated, it is similarly unlikely that the courts will overturn it. In short, the PSROs are probably here to stay. The question then becomes: What form will they assume? The answer, not surprisingly, is likely to depend heavily on two factors: Congressional budgeting, and the actions which HEW takes in its future attempts to implement the law.

The primary consideration, of course, is funding. The PSRO law could be left on the books while the PSROs and HEW's internal PSRO-related staff are forced to reduce their size and scope of operations. If this happens, implementation of the law would slow even further than its already turtlelike pace, and the PSRO law would become essentially a dead letter. PSRO-related litigation would, one expects, become similarly dormant. It is entirely possible that financial strangulation will in fact be the fate of the PSRO program. It will certainly happen if PSROs' opponents can prove that PSROs are failing to cut costs and/or improve quality, but it can happen just as easily if PSROs are perceived by Congress to be ineffective or counterproductive, even in the absence of proof.

To some extent, the onus rests on those, within HEW and elsewhere, who wish to preserve the PSRO program to develop and use a method of PSRO evaluation which is outcomes-related and can answer the question: Are PSROs having the effects they were designed to have? HEW's continued emphasis on process evaluation in the PSRO program (Are the PSROs spending too much money on their physician-reviewers? How many memoranda of understanding have been signed? etc.) can only lead to political disaster if it is not linked with an outcomes evaluation which can help Congress decide whether or not the program deserves continued support. What is crucial is that the evaluation be universal: to evaluate some groups and ignore others is to invite a challenge to the results on the grounds of statistical bias.

HEW's influence over the PSRO program's future is crucial in one other major area as well: regulation. (Here we will assume, for the sake of discussion, that adequate funding is obtained.) If HEW takes a "cautious" position in drafting regulations, the PSRO program may go forward without any serious legal challenge from the medical professions. If consumers' groups which might otherwise be interested were to decide as a result that the PSRO program is of sufficiently low visibility so that lawsuits would cost more than they are worth, a program acceptable to organized medicine could then be implemented. If, however, HEW drafts a more "aggressive" set of regulations, demanding extremely stringent review, litigation is more probable. It must be stated that, costs aside, HEW's best course might well be to risk litigation. If it drafts cautious regulations, it may emasculate the PSRO program when there is no legal necessity to do so, whereas if it drafts stringent regulations, the courts may well uphold its position.

The most probable areas of legal conflict, if HEW takes the latter position, may not necessarily be those of the greatest real concern to physicians and institutional administrators. The costs of complying with a review program, for instance, will not necessarily be of concern to the courts even if they are high enough to lead either a PSRO or a reviewed institution to break its reimbursement contract with the other party. Anti-PSRO litigation is more likely to focus on the issues of invasion of privacy and deprivation of the patients' asserted right to treatment—both of which are important, certainly, but neither of which would necessarily engender litigation if large sums of money were not also at stake.

The courts will emphasize these two issues because they are the areas in which the PSRO program is most vulnerable to attack, and because they are the areas in which the law is most unsettled. If PSRO's opponents wish to argue about costs or changes in the quality of medical care, their primary forum will have to be political—Congress or HEW— rather than legal.

If the courts are given the problem of determining the legality of any of the PSRO regulations, as it seems likely they will if the program continues, the litigants may well find that some decisions are rendered that neither side has foreseen or desires. It is probable, for example, that PSROs could find themselves labeled as agencies of the federal government as a result of litigation over HEW's regulations on the confidentiality of PSRO data, no matter who wins the case on the main question (to uphold or strike down the regulations). Or, to take another example, if there is litigation over the question of preadmission screening, the PSROs may well find that their ability to use coordinators rather than physician-reviewers in some or all phases of concurrent review could be severely limited by the courts.

It is almost as risky to predict courts' decisions as it is to predict the political future of a federal program: at best, the predictor can be fairly sure but never certain. One purpose of this review is to warn again that the law has a momentum of its own, and that those who go to court to battle over issue x (e.g., the heavy cost impact of preadmission screening) may find the court making its decision on the basis of issue y (e.g., preadmission screening's denial of the patients' constitutionally protected right to medical treatment) and incidentally deciding issue z (e.g., the review coordinators' right/ability to make "medical" decisions during preadmission review) in order to reach the point at which issue y

can be decided. What the PSRO program will look like, once the dust has settled, cannot be predicted.

Other Review Programs

Obviously enough, a "private" peer review organization that does review for a state Medicaid agency can be defined by the courts as a "governmental" agency just as easily as can a PSRO that does review for the federal government; all of the same common-law considerations will apply to both, and while statutory and constitutional considerations differ for the public and private groups, the trend is probably towards increasing convergence in the way the courts treat both types. Even at the present time, hospital-based review groups that operate purely internally, while they may not have to worry about privacy laws to the same extent as do more clearly "governmental" organizations, may also have to concern themselves with constitutional due process standards, as more and more courts are defining hospitals themselves as "quasi-governmental."

Unlike PSROs, private and state-connected review groups will have to worry about such things as state privacy statutes; as they are not creatures of the federal government, the state and private groups will not be able to rely on the argument that federal law preempts state statutes. On the other hand, there may be an equitable trade-off: while federal statutes have the reputation, at least among some lawyers, of being better-written than most state statutes, and therefore preferable, state regulatory processes may be more responsive than the federal regulatory system.

One other possible difference between PSROs and the nonfederal review groups bears note: insurance. PSROs may or may not be defined as "agencies" for purposes of the Federal Tort Claims Act, and if they are they may therefore be able to avoid having to obtain coverage against routine torts. For the nonfederal groups the reality is that there are few alternatives to private insurance to cover the possible misdeeds of review group employees, state immunity laws being, as they are, limited in scope and legally untested. It can be hypothesized that such insurance may be scarce and expensive for the same reasons that have plagued malpractice insurance: insufficient actuarial experience, a restricted group of purchasers, and the possibility of increasing involvement in litigation.

Where is legal trouble most likely to occur for the non-PSRO review groups? If past experience is any guide, these organizations are more likely to become involved in routine malpractice cases than in major constitutional litigation (over, for example, the extent of patients' privacy rights). Of course, past experience may be no guide. Because most of the private and state-connected review groups are in fact very much like PSROs, they may be hit by a "spill-over" effect when and if dissatisfied physicians, hospitals, and patients realize that many of the arguments that win anti-PSRO litigation can win against the other groups as well.

Prediction in this area, as in others, is extremely risky. Again it must be reiterated that ultimately the facts and arguments which will be most hotly contested are not necessarily those of the greatest initial interest to the participants. Physicians may react adversely to a review group's creation of treatment profiles, but if they live in a state in which the laws on physician-patient privilege have consistently been interpreted as being for the benefit of the patient rather than the physician, they may find that their only legal precedent is that which they create for themselves, a risky business at best.

ALTERNATIVES

The word "alternatives" here involves two concepts: alternatives to present review systems, and alternatives to present review law. If anything is certain, it is that both the systems and the law will change in the coming years. It is the manner in which they will change that is uncertain. Will there be an economic depression in the medical industry? If so, will the prospect of tight money lead to the development of more sophisticated review systems designed to improve the allocation of scarce medical resources? Or will the economic crunch lead people to junk the review systems because they divert money that would, or at least could, otherwise be used to provide treatment to patients? If there is prosperity, will review programs be ignored as unnecessary? Or will they achieve new support because of their utility in improving quality?

If the future of the review programs is uncertain, the possible nature of their potential substitutes is an enigma of the worst sort. Some suggestions have been made, however, and they include the following:

- *Changes in Insurance Coverage.* Some have suggested that federal and private insurance packages should be redesigned to provide more reimbursement for preventive and primary care and less for emergency, acute, and chronic care. While it is probable that such redesigning would have a beneficial long-range effect (if the assumption holds true that patients will seek out care for which the third party pays in preference to care for which they pay directly), the short-range problems could be substantial. A decrease in federal coverage of the costs of acute-care hospitalization would be politically unwelcome, and the private carriers claim that such policies are virtually unsaleable: there is no consumer demand for policies which cover the cheap office visit and leave the patient to pay a substantial proportion of the expensive hospitalization. On the other hand, if peer review proves ineffective, a reduction in the outlay for certain types of expensive treatments may be the only immediately feasible alternative.

• *Expansion of the HMOs.* Health Maintenance Organizations appear at this time to provide at least adequate medical service for their patients at lower cost than do fee-for-service physicians using traditional referral patterns. It has been suggested that if HMOs were to expand, the total cost to society of providing health care would be reduced. However, there are those who argue that one of the major factors contributing to the apparently lower cost of care within HMOs is that the HMOs ordinarily insure and treat the healthiest segment of society: the young and middle-aged middle class. Whether HMO costs would rise to present fee-for-service levels even if the HMOs included an average number of the elderly and chronically ill is not yet known, but it is certainly possible to argue that even if the nature of the covered population were to change, the HMOs would still come out ahead financially, as they can regulate their costs by limiting practitioners' salaries, increasing their use of physicians' assistants, or changing their hospital-affiliation agreements when such agreements exist. At the moment, however, HMO expansion is not a viable alternative to peer review as a cost-cutting mechanism, as the government can encourage HMO development but cannot force physicians to join, and there is considerable opposition to salaried practice among many members of the medical profession.

• *Creation of a Federally-controlled National Health Service.* Obviously, this is the least feasible alternative of all. All the political considerations that make HMOs obnoxious to physicians apply with even greater force to the prospect of a salaried, or at least reimbursement-controlled, national health service. Furthermore, it is not known whether fully "socialized" medicine would be acceptable to the majority of American citizens, and it is certainly possible to hypothesize that there exists a significant segment of the population to whom nonprivate medical care would be anathema. We raise this possibility only because it exists as a very real long-term consequence of continued cost increase in medicine. If peer review and/or other, less drastic, cost- and quality-control mechanisms have insufficient impact, and if federal national health insurance effectively drives private payment into extinction, we may well find that we have developed a medical payment system which in effect forces the government to exert drastic *a priori* financial control of the health industry.

It should be clear that all three of the above alternatives differ from peer review in one significant aspect: decisions are made about care "generically" and before it is rendered. Where peer review makes payment and other decisions only after an individual physician-patient encounter has been initiated, the alternatives do not necessarily have that kind of flexibility. A physician in an HMO cannot get that HMO to pay for his patient's dental care if the HMO doesn't cover dental care, even if the physician is convinced that appropriate dental treatment is the one thing most likely to cure his patient's headaches. If a patient's health insurance covers no more than ten days of nursing home care and the patient has no alternate source of funds, the chronically ill patient's physician may have to develop a less-desirable treatment plan in order to get any care to the patient at all. To the extent that peer review operates within the confines of existing insurance reimbursement packages, whether federal or private, it suffers the same disabilities; but the advantage of concurrent peer review is that by limiting reimbursement for unnecessary covered care it may free money for care which could not otherwise be covered. In short, it is a theoretically better method of resource allocation. If its costs can be kept within acceptable limits, it is probably preferable to most of the alternatives that have been suggested so far.

So much for the alternatives to peer review. What about alternatives to peer review law? Surely there must be some physicians who, having read their way through Chapters 4 through 8, and arriving here at last, may ask themselves, "How did we get involved in this swamp?"

The lawyer's answer might be, "People who become involved with peer review programs, like people everywhere, have interests—and rights—which they may wish to preserve or assert, and resorting to the courts and Congress is the best method of preserving or creating rights that American society has been able to come up with so far." The answer may be true as far as it goes, but it may be that the law—as it has periodically throughout history—is becoming an object of increasing fearfulness and suspicion to the average citizen, who sees in its expense, delay, and convoluted arguments more that confuses than that comforts. If this is the case, it is quite possible that simpler new procedures and possibly even new types of courts will be devised, with the "court" —or whatever it is called—given the freedom to create its own law as it goes along. Such developments, alas, will probably arrive, if they arrive at all, too late to be of any use to PSROs or other peer review groups. In short, there is apparently no realistic alternative to the present legal system available. Specific laws may change; courts may create precedent or break it; Congress and the state legislatures may modify or even repeal statutes; federal and state executive agencies may issue any number of regulations. In all cases, however, the changes will be made within the context of the present legal system and defined by their relationship to present law. How did we get involved in this swamp? We are involved because it's there, the solutions are on the far side, and we have to cross it if we don't want to drown.

NOTES

1. At the time this book was written, there were only two reported cases: Assn. of Am. Phys. & Surg. v. Weinberger, 395 F. Supp 125 (1975) and Texas Med. Assn. v. Mathews, 408 F. Supp 303 (1976). The California delegation case was settled, and the Massachusetts confidentiality case has not been argued.

The PSRO program has received mention in two related cases: Mt. Sinai Hosp. of Greater Miami v. Weinberger, 376 F. Supp 1099 (1974), 517 F.2d 329 (1975) and Szekely v. Florida Med. Assn, 517 F.2d 345 (1975), in which a federally funded non-PSRO peer review program was attacked, *inter alia,* for overlapping the PSRO's mandate. The courts were not impressed.

Appendix A

Sources of Law

American law, broadly speaking, represents a composite of three basic types of law—judicial, legislative and regulatory. It is important to note that American law operates on two distinct planes: federal and state. Federal law takes precedence over state law in situations where these two sets of laws conflict, according to the principles laid out in the supremacy clause of the U.S. Constitution.

1. The Judiciary

Judicial law constitutes that set of legal principles developed by the judiciary arising out of specific disputes placed before a court. Common law is a term often used to describe this case law (as originated in England and adopted and expanded in the American legal system). A specific determination rendered by a judge establishes the law not only in that given case but in other similar cases where the court has jurisdiction.

Even if a case is in the same court system, however, one court does not often set precedent for another. For example, a federal court of appeals in the first circuit is not bound by a decision in another federal court of appeals, although it is strongly influenced by other federal appellate decisions. A decision sets precedent only for the courts below it. Therefore, a decision by the Second Circuit Court of Appeals is binding on all District Courts in the second circuit, but can be overturned by a later Second Circuit Court of Appeals decision or a U.S. Supreme Court decision. A decision by the Massachusetts Supreme Judicial Court is binding on the Massachusetts Superior Court (trial level) and Appeals Court (first appellate level) but can be overturned by the Supreme Judicial Court or U.S. Supreme Court. A decision by a trial court is never binding.

Court decisions are "reported" in a series of official and unofficial publications. For example, U.S. Supreme Court decisions can be found in the official United States Reports and the unofficial Supreme Court Reports; decisions of many states' highest courts can be found in official state publications (e.g., Ohio Reports; Massachusetts Reports; New York Reports, Second Series) and unofficial "regional reporters."

2. The Legislature

Statutory law is that body of law enacted by a legislature, either federal or state, and subject to judicial interpretation. Legislation acts as the legal framework within which government-sanctioned public affairs are conducted.

There are two general types of statutes: public laws and private laws. Private laws are usually designed to affect the rights of a small group of known people, such as a group of prisoners of war who are being prosecuted by the Internal Revenue Service for failure to pay taxes or file tax reports during their captivity. Private laws name the persons they affect, and in some states are not routinely published. Public laws affect the population at large, and are always published, often in two forms: chronological and codified. For example, the PSRO law can be found in the federal Statutes at Large as Section 249F of PL 92-603 (Public Law #603 of the 92nd Congress) and is codified in the U.S. Code as sections 1320c thru 1320c-19 of Title 42 (42 U.S.C. §§1320c—1320c-19).

3. The Executive

Regulatory law is derived from legislation, for many statutes contain specific provisions granting power to administrative agencies to issue regulations implementing a particular law. It is often difficult (and politically unfeasible) at the time of passage of legislation to be specific concerning details of implementation. Regulatory law thus places great power in the hands of the secretary of an administrative agency, who can through regulations shape the overall effect of a piece of legislation.

Regulations are only as strong as the statutes on which they are based, so a court decision that invalidates a statute also invalidates regulations promulgated under that statute's authority. A court can also find a specific regulation illegal or unconstitutional even when its statute is constitutional.

Federal regulations are published chronologically in the *Federal Register* and codified in the *Code of Federal Regulations*. State regulations are often published randomly (or not at all) by whichever state agency promulgates them, and are rarely codified. Despite their being difficult to locate, such regulations are nevertheless law, and must be obeyed just as statutes and court decisions are obeyed.

Appendix B
PSRO Law—P.L. 92-603

Public Law 92-603
92nd Congress, H. R. 1
October 30, 1972

𝔄n 𝔄ct

86 STAT. 1329

To amend the Social Security Act, and for other purposes.

Be it enacted by the Senate and House of Representatives of the United States of America in Congress assembled, That this Act, with the following table of contents, may be cited as the "Social Security Amendments of 1972". Social Security Amendments of 1972.

"TITLE XI—GENERAL PROVISIONS"

and inserting in lieu thereof

"TITLE XI—GENERAL PROVISIONS AND PROFESSIONAL STANDARDS REVIEW

"PART A—GENERAL PROVISIONS"

(b) Title XI of such Act is further amended by adding the following:

"PART B—PROFESSIONAL STANDARDS REVIEW

"DECLARATION OF PURPOSE

"SEC. 1151. In order to promote the effective, efficient, and economical delivery of health care services of proper quality for which payment may be made (in whole or in part) under this Act and in recognition of the interests of patients, the public, practitioners, and providers in improved health care services, it is the purpose of this part to assure, through the application of suitable procedures of professional standards review, that the services for which payment may be made under the Social Security Act will conform to appropriate professional standards for the provision of health care and that payment for such services will be made—

217

Pub. Law 92-603   **October 30, 1972**

"(1) only when, and to the extent, medically necessary, as determined in the exercise of reasonable limits of professional discretion; and

"(2) in the case of services provided by a hospital or other health care facility on an inpatient basis, only when and for such period as such services cannot, consistent with professionally recognized health care standards, effectively be provided on an outpatient basis or more economically in an inpatient health care facility of a different type, as determined in the exercise of reasonable limits of professional discretion.

"DESIGNATION OF PROFESSIONAL STANDARDS REVIEW ORGANIZATIONS

"SEC. 1152. (a) The Secretary shall (1) not later than January 1, 1974, establish throughout the United States appropriate areas with respect to which Professional Standards Review Organizations may be designated, and (2) at the earliest practicable date after designation of an area enter into an agreement with a qualified organization whereby such an organization shall be conditionally designated as the Professional Standards Review Organization for such area. If, on the basis of its performance during such period of conditional designation, the Secretary determines that such organization is capable of fulfilling, in a satisfactory manner, the obligations and requirements for a Professional Standards Review Organization under this part, he shall enter into an agreement with such organization designating it as the Professional Standards Review Organization for such area.

"Qualified or-
ganization."

"(b) For purposes of subsection (a), the term 'qualified organization' means—

"(1) when used in connection with any area—

"(A) an organization (i) which is a nonprofit professional association (or a component organization thereof), (ii) which is composed of licensed doctors of medicine or osteopathy engaged in the practice of medicine or surgery in such area, (iii) the membership of which includes a substantial proportion of all such physicians in such area, (iv) which is organized in a manner which makes available professional competence to review health care services of the types and kinds with respect to which Professional Standards Review Organizations have review responsibilities under this part, (v) the membership of which is voluntary and open to all doctors of medicine or osteopathy licensed to engage in the practice of medicine or surgery in such area without requirement of membership in or payment of dues to any organized medical society or association, and (vi) which does not restrict the eligibility of any member for service as an officer of the Professional Standards Review Organization or eligibility for and assignment to duties of such Professional Standards Review Organization, or, subject to subsection (c)(i),

"(B) such other public, nonprofit private, or other agency or organization, which the Secretary determines, in accordance with criteria prescribed by him in regulations, to be of professional competence and otherwise suitable; and

"(2) an organization which the Secretary, on the basis of his examination and evaluation of a formal plan submitted to him by the association, agency, or organization (as well as on the basis of other relevant data and information), finds to be willing to perform and capable of performing, in an effective, timely, and objective manner and at reasonable cost, the duties, functions, and

October 30, 1972   Pub. Law 92-603
                                                          86 STAT. 1431

activities of a Professional Standards Review Organization required by or pursuant to this part.

"(c) (1) The Secretary shall not enter into any agreement under this part under which there is designated as the Professional Standards Review Organization for any area any organization other than an organization referred to in subsection (b) (1) (A) prior to January 1, 1976, nor after such date, unless, in such area, there is no organization referred to in subsection (b) (1) (A) which meets the conditions specified in subsection (b) (2).

"(2) Whenever the Secretary shall have entered into an agreement under this part under which there is designated as the Professional Standards Review Organization for any area any organization other than an organization referred to in subsection (b) (1) (A), he shall not renew such agreements with such organization if he determines that—

"(A) there is in such area an organization referred to in subsection (b) (1) (A) which (i) has not been previously designated as a Professional Standards Review Organization, and (ii) is willing to enter into an agreement under this part under which such organization would be designated as the Professional Standards Review Organization for such area;

"(B) such organization meets the conditions specified in subsection (b) (2) ; and

"(C) the designation of such organization as the Professional Standards Review Organization for such area is anticipated to result in substantial improvement in the performance in such area of the duties and functions required of such organizations under this part.

"(d) Any such agreement under this part with an organization (other than an agreement established pursuant to section 1154) shall be for a term of 12 months; except that, prior to the expiration of such term such agreement may be terminated—

Agreement expiration, prior termination. Post, p. 1432.

"(1) by the organization at such time and upon such notice to the Secretary as may be prescribed in regulations (except that notice of more than 3 months may not be required) ; or

"(2) by the Secretary at such time and upon such reasonable notice to the organization as may be prescribed in regulations, but only after the Secretary has determined (after providing such organization with an opportunity for a formal hearing on the matter) that such organization is not substantially complying with or effectively carrying out the provisions of such agreement.

"(e) In order to avoid duplication of functions and unnecessary review and control activities, the Secretary is authorized to waive any or all of the review, certification, or similar activities otherwise required under or pursuant to any provision of this Act (other than this part) where he finds, on the basis of substantial evidence of the effective performance of review and control activities by Professional Standards Review Organizations, that the review, certification, and similar activities otherwise so required are not needed for the provision of adequate review and control.

Waiver.

"(f)(1) In the case of agreements entered into prior to January 1, 1976, under this part under which any organization is designated as the Professional Standards Review Organization for any area, the Secretary shall, prior to entering into any such agreement with any organization for any area, inform (under regulations of the Secretary) the doctors of medicine or osteopathy who are in active practice in such area of the Secretary's intention to enter into such an agreement with such organization.

Agreement notice.

Pub. Law 92-603   - 104 -   October 30, 1972

"(2) If, within a reasonable period of time following the serving of such notice, more than 10 per centum of such doctors object to the Secretary's entering into such an agreement with such organization on the ground that such organization is not representative of doctors in such area, the Secretary shall conduct a poll of such doctors to determine whether or not such organization is representative of such doctors in such area. If more than 50 per centum of the doctors responding to such poll indicate that such organization is not representative of such doctors in such area the Secretary shall not enter into such an agreement with such organization.

"REVIEW PENDING DESIGNATION OF PROFESSIONAL STANDARDS REVIEW ORGANIZATION

"Sec. 1153. Pending the assumption by a Professional Standards Review Organization for any area, of full review responsibility, and pending a demonstration of capacity for improved review effort with respect to matters involving the provision of health care services in such area for which payment (in whole or in part) may be made, under this Act, any review with respect to such services which has not been designated by the Secretary as the full responsibility of such organization, shall be reviewed in the manner otherwise provided for under law.

"TRIAL PERIOD FOR PROFESSIONAL STANDARDS REVIEW ORGANIZATIONS

"Sec. 1154. (a) The Secretary shall initially designate an organization as a Professional Standards Review Organization for any area on a conditional basis with a view to determining the capacity of such organization to perform the duties and functions imposed under this part on Professional Standards Review Organizations. Such designation may not be made prior to receipt from such organization and approval by the Secretary of a formal plan for the orderly assumption and implementation of the responsibilities of the Professional Standards Review Organization under this part.

Plan, approval.

Duties.

"(b) During any such trial period (which may not exceed 24 months), the Secretary may require a Professional Standards Review Organization to perform only such of the duties and functions required under this part of Professional Standards Review Organization as he determines such organization to be capable of performing. The number and type of such duties shall, during the trial period, be progressively increased as the organization becomes capable of added responsibility so that, by the end of such period, such organization shall be considered a qualified organization only if the Secretary finds that it is substantially carrying out in a satisfactory manner, the activities and functions required of Professional Standards Review Organizations under this part with respect to the review of health care services provided or ordered by physicians and other practitioners and institutional and other health care facilities, agencies, and organizations. Any of such duties and functions not performed by such organization during such period shall be performed in the manner and to the extent otherwise provided for under law.

Termination, notice.

"(c) Any agreement under which any organization is conditionally designated as the Professional Standards Review Organization for any area may be terminated by such organization upon 90 days notice to the Secretary or by the Secretary upon 90 days notice to such organization.

October 30, 1972   - 105 -   Pub. Law 92-603   <u>86 STAT. 1433</u>

"DUTIES AND FUNCTIONS OF PROFESSIONAL STANDARDS REVIEW
ORGANIZATIONS

"SEC. 1155. (a) (1) Notwithstanding any other provision of law, but
consistent with the provisions of this part, it shall (subject to the provisions of subsection (g)) be the duty and function of each Professional Standards Review Organization for any area to assume, at the
earliest date practicable, responsibility for the review of the professional activities in such area of physicians and other health care practitioners and institutional and noninstitutional providers of health
care services in the provision of health care services and items for
which payment may be made (in whole or in part) under this Act for
the purpose of determining whether—
    "(A) such services and items are or were medically necessary,
    "(B) the quality of such services meets professionally recog-
nized standards of health care; and
    "(C) in case such services and items are proposed to be pro-
vided in a hospital or other health care facility on an inpatient
basis, such services and items could, consistent with the provision
of appropriate medical care, be effectively provided on an out-
patient basis or more economically in an inpatient health care
facility of a different type.
    "(2) Each Professional Standards Review Organization shall have
the authority to determine, in advance. in the case of—
    "(A) any elective admission to a hospital, or other health care
facility, or
    "(B) any other health care service which will consist of
extended or costly courses of treatment,
whether such service, if provided, or if provided by a particular health
care practitioner or by a particular hospital or other health care
facility, organization, or agency, would meet the criteria specified in
clauses (A) and (C) of paragraph (1).
    "(3) Each Professional Standards Review Organization shall, in
accordance with regulations of the Secretary, determine and publish,
from time to time, the types and kinds of cases (whether by type of
health care or diagnosis involved, or whether in terms of other relevant criteria relating to the provision of health care services) with
respect to which such organization will, in order most effectively to
carry out the purposes of this part, exercise the authority conferred
upon it under paragraph (2).   *Case criteria, publication.*
    "(4) Each Professional Standards Review Organization shall be
responsible for the arranging for the maintenance of and the regular
review of profiles of care and services received and provided with
respect to patients, utilizing to the greatest extent practicable in such
patient profiles, methods of coding which wi l provide maximum confidentiality as to patient identity and assure objective evaluation consistent with the purposes of this part. Profiles shall also be regularly
reviewed on an ongoing basis with respect to each health care practitioner and provider to determine whether the care and services
ordered or rendered are consistent with the criteria specified in clauses
(A), (B), and (C) of paragraph (1).   *Patient profiles, maintenance and review.*
    "(5) Physicians assigned responsibility for the review of hospital
care may be only those having active hospital staff privileges in at
least one of the participating hospitals in the area served by the Professional Standards Review Organization and (except as may be otherwise provided under subsection (e) (1) of this section) such physicians
ordinarily should not be responsible for, but may participate in the
review of care and services provided in any hospital in which such
physicians have active staff privileges.   *Hospital care, physician review.*

"(6) No physician shall be permitted to review—

"(A) health care services provided to a patient if he was directly or indirectly involved in providing such services, or

"(B) health care services provided in or by an institution, organization, or agency, if he or any member of his family has, directly or indirectly, any financial interest in such institution, organization, or agency.

Physician's family.

For purposes of this paragraph, a physician's family includes only his spouse (other than a spouse who is legally separated from him under a decree of divorce or separate maintenance), children (including legally adopted children), grandchildren, parents, and grandparents.

"(b) To the extent necessary or appropriate for the proper performance of its duties and functions, the Professional Standards Review Organization serving any area is authorized in accordance with regulations prescribed by the Secretary to—

"(1) make arrangements to utilize the services of persons who are practitioners of or specialists in the various areas of medicine (including dentistry), or other types of health care, which persons shall, to the maximum extent practicable, be individuals engaged in the practice of their profession within the area served by such organization;

"(2) undertake such professional inquiry either before or after, or both before and after, the provision of services with respect to which such organization has a responsibility for review under subsection (a) (1);

"(3) examine the pertinent records of any practitioner or provider of health care services providing services with respect to which such organization has a responsibility for review under subsection (a) (1); and

"(4) inspect the facilities in which care is rendered or services provided (which are located in such area) of any practitioner or provider.

"(c) No Professional Standards Review Organization shall utilize the services of any individual who is not a duly licensed doctor of medicine or osteopathy to make final determinations in accordance with its duties and functions under this part with respect to the professional conduct of any other duly licensed doctor of medicine or osteopathy, or any act performed by any duly licensed doctor of medicine or osteopathy in the exercise of his profession.

"(d) In order to familiarize physicians with the review functions and activities of Professional Standards Review Organizations and to promote acceptance of such functions and activities by physicians, patients, and other persons, each Professional Standards Review Organization, in carrying out its review responsibilities, shall (to the maximum extent consistent with the effective and timely performance of its duties and functions)—

"(1) encourage all physicians practicing their profession in the area served by such Organization to participate as reviewers in the review activities of such Organizations;

"(2) provide rotating physician membership of review committees on an extensive and continuing basis;

"(3) assure that membership on review committees have the broadest representation feasible in terms of the various types of practice in which physicians engage in the area served by such Organization; and

"(4) utilize, whenever appropriate, medical periodicals and similar publications to publicize the functions and activities of Professional Standards Review Organizations.

October 30, 1972   Pub. Law 92-603 86 STAT. 1435

"(e)(1) Each Professional Standards Review Organization shall Review committee
utilize the services of, and accept the findings of, the review com- tees.
mittees of a hospital or other operating health care facility or organization located in the area served by such organization, but only when
and only to the extent and only for such time that such committees in
such hospital or other operating health care facility or organization
have demonstrated to the satisfaction of such organization their
capacity effectively and in timely fashion to review activities in such
hospital or other operating health care facility or organization
(including the medical necessity of admissions, types and extent of
services ordered, and lengths of stay) so as to aid in accomplishing
the purposes and responsibilities described in subsection (a)(1), except
where the Secretary disapproves, for good cause, such acceptance.
"(2) The Secretary may prescribe regulations to carry out the pro- Regulations.
visions of this subsection.
"(f)(1) An agreement entered into under this part between the Agreement re-
Secretary and any organization under which such organization is quirements.
designated as the Professional Standards Review Organization for
any area shall provide that such organization will—
  "(A) perform such duties and functions and assume such
  responsibilities and comply with such other requirements as may
  be required by this part or under regulations of the Secretary
  promulgated to carry out the provisions of this part; and
  "(B) collect such data relevant to its functions and such information and keep and maintain such records in such form as
  the Secretary may require to carry out the purposes of this part
  and to permit access to and use of any such records as the Secretary may require for such purposes.
"(2) Any such agreement with an organization under this part shall
provide that the Secretary make payments to such organization equal
to the amount of expenses reasonably and necessarily incurred, as
determined by the Secretary, by such organization in carrying out or
preparing to carry out the duties and functions required by such
agreement.
"(g) Notwithstanding any other provision of this part, the responsibility for review of health care services of any Professional
Standards Review Organization shall be the review of health care
services provided by or in institutions, unless such Organization shall
have made a request to the Secretary that it be charged with the
duty and function of reviewing other health care services and the
Secretary shall have approved such request.

"NORMS OF HEALTH CARE SERVICES FOR VARIOUS ILLNESSES OR HEALTH
CONDITIONS

"SEC. 1156. (a) Each Professional Standards Review Organization
shall apply professionally developed norms of care, diagnosis, and
treatment based upon typical patterns of practice in its regions
(including typical lengths-of-stay for institutional care by age and
diagnosis) as principal points of evaluation and review. The National
Professional Standards Review Council and the Secretary shall provide such technical assistance to the organization as will be helpful
in utilizing and applying such norms of care, diagnosis, and treatment.
Where the actual norms of care, diagnosis, and treatment in a Professional Standards Review Organization area are significantly different
from professionally developed regional norms of care, diagnosis, and

86 STAT, 1436   Pub. Law 92-603   October 30, 1972

treatment approved for comparable conditions, the Professional Standards Review Organization concerned shall be so informed, and in the event that appropriate consultation and discussion indicate reasonable basis for usage of other norms in the area concerned, the Professional Standards Review Organization may apply such norms in such area as are approved by the National Professional Standards Review Council.

"(b) Such norms with respect to treatment for particular illnesses or health conditions shall include (in accordance with regulations of the Secretary)—

"(1) the types and extent of the health care services which, taking into account differing, but acceptable, modes of treatment and methods of organizing and delivering care are considered within the range of appropriate diagnosis and treatment of such illness or health condition, consistent with professionally recognized and accepted patterns of care;

"(2) the type of health care facility which is considered, consistent with such standards, to be the type in which health care services which are medically appropriate for such illness or condition can most economically be provided.

Preparation and distribution of data.

"(c)(1) The National Professional Standards Review Council shall provide for the preparation and distribution, to each Professional Standards Review Organization and to each other agency or person performing review functions with respect to the provision of health care services under this Act, of appropriate materials indicating the regional norms to be utilized pursuant to this part. Such data concerning norms shall be reviewed and revised from time to time. The approval of the National Professional Standards Review Council of norms of care, diagnosis, and treatment shall be based on its analysis of appropriate and adequate data.

"(2) Each review organization, agency, or person referred to in paragraph (1) shall utilize the norms developed under this section as a principal point of evaluation and review for determining, with respect to any health care services which have been or are proposed to be provided, whether such care and services are consistent with the criteria

Ante, p. 1433.

specified in section 1155(a)(1).

"(d)(1) Each Professional Standards Review Organization shall—

"(A) in accordance with regulations of the Secretary, specify the appropriate points in time after the admission of a patient for inpatient care in a health care institution, at which the physician attending such patient shall execute a certification stating that further inpatient care in such institution will be medically necessary effectively to meet the health care needs of such patient; and

"(B) require that there be included in any such certification with respect to any patient such information as may be necessary to enable such organization properly to evaluate the medical necessity of the further institutional health care recommended by the physician executing such certification.

"(2) The points in time at which any such certification will be required (usually, not later than the 50th percentile of lengths-of-stay for patients in similar age groups with similar diagnoses) shall be consistent with and based on professionally developed norms of care and treatment and data developed with respect to length of stay in health care institutions of patients having various illnesses, injuries, or health conditions, and requiring various types of health care services or procedures.

October 30, 1972   Pub. Law 92-603   86 STAT. 1437

"SUBMISSION OF REPORTS BY PROFESIONAL STANDARDS REVIEW
ORGANIZATIONS

"Sec. 1157. If, in discharging its duties and functions under this
part, any Professional Standards Review Organization determines
that any health care practitioner or any hospital, or other health
care facility, agency, or organization has violated any of the obligations imposed by section 1160, such organization shall report the   Post, p. 1438.
matter to the Statewide Professional Standards Review Council for
the State in which such organization is located together with the
recommendations of such Organization as to the action which should
be taken with respect to the matter. Any Statewide Professional
Standards Review Council receiving any such report and recommendation shall review the same and promptly transmit such report
and recommendation to the Secretary together with any additional
comments or recommendations thereon as it deems appropriate. The
Secretary may utilize a Professional Standards Review Organization,
in lieu of a program review team as specified in sections 1862 and 1866,   79 Stat. 325;
for purposes of subparagraph (C) of section 1862(d)(1) and sub-   81 Stat. 846.
paragraph (F) of section 1866(b)(2).   42 USC 1395y,
                                                        1395oo.
                                                        Ante, p. 1408,

"REQUIREMENT OF REVIEW APPROVAL AS CONDITION OF PAYMENT OF CLAIMS   Ante, p. 1409.

"Sec. 1158. (a) Except as provided for in section 1159, no Federal
funds appropriated under any title of this Act (other than title V)   81 Stat. 921.
for the provision of health care services or items shall be used (directly   42 USC 701.
or indirectly) for the payment, under such title or any program established pursuant thereto, of any claim for the provision of such services
or items, unless the Secretary, pursuant to regulation determines that
the claimant is without fault if—
     "(1) the provision of such services or items is subject to review
under this part by any Professional Standards Review Organization, or other agency; and
     "(2) such organization or other agency has, in the proper exer-
cise of its duties and functions under or consistent with the
purposes of this part, disapproved of the services or items giving
rise to such claim, and has notified the practitioner or provider
who provided or proposed to provide such services or items and
the individual who would receive or was proposed to receive such
services or items of its disapproval of the provision of such
services or items.
   "(b) Whenever any Professional Standards Review Organization,
in the discharge of its duties and functions as specified by or pursuant
to this part, disapproves of any health care services or items furnished
or to be furnished by any practitioner or provider, such organization
shall, after notifying the practitioner, provider, or other organization
or agency of its disapproval in accordance with subsection (a),
promptly notify the agency or organization having responsibility for
acting upon claims for payment for or on account of such services or
items.

"HEARINGS AND REVIEW BY SECRETARY

"Sec. 1159. (a) Any beneficiary or recipient who is entitled to benefits under this Act (other than title V) or a provider or practitioner
who is dissatisfied with a determination with respect to a claim made
by a Professional Standards Review Organization in carrying out its
responsibilities for the review of professional activities in accordance
with paragraphs (1) and (2) of section 1155(a) shall, after being   Ante, p. 1433.

Pub. Law 92-603 October 30, 1972

notified of such determination, be entitled to a reconsideration thereof by the Professional Standards Review Organization and, where the Professional Standards Review Organization reaffirms such determination in a State which has established a Statewide Professional Standards Review Council, and where the matter in controversy is $100 or more, such determination shall be reviewed by professional members of such Council and, if the Council so determined, revised.

"(b) Where the determination of the Statewide Professional Standards Review Council is adverse to the beneficiary or recipient (or, in the absence of such Council in a State and where the matter in controversy is $100 or more), such beneficiary or recipient shall be entitled to a hearing thereon by the Secretary to the same extent as is provided

53 Stat. 1368,
42 USC 405. in section 205(b), and, where the amount in controversy is $1,000 or more, to judicial review of the Secretary's final decision after such hearing as is provided in section 205(g). The Secretary will render a decision only after appropriate professional consultation on the matter.

"(c) Any review or appeals provided under this section shall be in lieu of any review, hearing, or appeal under this Act with respect to the same issue.

"OBLIGATIONS OF HEALTH CARE PRACTITIONERS AND PROVIDERS OF HEALTH CARE SERVICES; SANCTIONS AND PENALTIES; HEARINGS AND REVIEW

"SEC. 1160. (a)(1) It shall be the obligation of any health care practitioner and any other person (including a hospital or other health care facility, organization, or agency) who provides health care services for which payment may be made (in whole or in part) under this Act, to assure that services or items ordered or provided by such practitioner or person to beneficiaries and recipients under this Act—

"(A) will be provided only when, and to the extent, medically necessary; and

"(B) will be of a quality which meets professionally recognized standards of health care: and

"(C) will be supported by evidence of such medical necessity and quality in such form and fashion and at such time as may reasonably be required by the Professional Standards Review Organization in the exercise of its duties and responsibilities:

and it shall be the obligation of any health care practitioner in ordering, authorizing. directing, or arranging for the provision by any other person (including a hospital or other health care facility, organization, or agency), of health care services for any patient of such practitioner, to exercise his professional responsibility with a view to assuring (to the extent of his influence or control over such patient, such person, or the provision of such services) that such services or items will be provided—

"(D) only when, and to the extent, medically necessary; and

"(E) will be of a quality which meets professionally recognized standards of health care.

"(2) Each health care practitioner. and each hospital or other provider of health care services. shall have an obligation, within reasonable limits of professional discretion, not to take any action, in the exercise of his profession (in the case of any health care practitioner), or in the conduct of its business (in the case of any hospital or other such provider), which would authorize any individual to be admitted as an inpatient in or to continue as an inpatient in any hospital or other health care facility unless—

October 30, 1972   **Pub. Law 92-603** 86 STAT. 1439

"(A) inpatient care is determined by such practitioner and by such hospital or other provider, consistent with professionally recognized health care standards, to be medically necessary for the proper care of such individual; and

"(B)(i) the inpatient care required by such individual cannot, consistent with such standards, be provided more economically in a health care facility of a different type; or

"(ii) (in the case of a patient who requires care which can, consistent with such standards, be provided more economically in a health care facility of a different type) there is, in the area in which such individual is located, no such facility or no such facility which is available to provide care to such individual at the time when care is needed by him.

"(b)(1) If after reasonable notice and opportunity for discussion Report and with the practitioner or provider concerned, any Professional Stand- recommenda-ards Review Organization submits a report and recommendations to tions. the Secretary pursuant to section 1157 (which report and recom- Ante, p. 1437. mendations shall be submitted through the Statewide Professional Standards Review Council, if such Council has been established, which shall promptly transmit such report and recommendations together with any additional comments and recommendations thereon as it deems appropriate) and if the Secretary determines that such practitioner or provider, in providing health care services over which such organization has review responsibility and for which payment (in whole or in part) may be made under this Act has—

"(A) by failing, in a substantial number of cases, substantially to comply with any obligation imposed on him under subsection (a), or

"(B) by grossly and flagrantly violating any such obligation in one or more instances,

demonstrated an unwillingness or a lack of ability substantially to comply with such obligations, he (in addition to any other sanction provided under law) may exclude (permanently for such period as the Secretary may prescribe) such practitioner or provider from eligibility to provide such services on a reimbursable basis.

"(2) A determination made by the Secretary under this subsection shall be effective at such time and upon such reasonable notice to the public and to the person furnishing the services involved as may be specified in regulations. Such determination shall be effective with respect to services furnished to an individual on or after the effective date of such determination (except that in the case of institutional health care services such determination shall be effective in the manner provided in title XVIII with respect to terminations of provider 79 Stat. 291. agreements), and shall remain in effect until the Secretary finds and 42 USC 1395. gives reasonable notice to the public that the basis for such determination has been removed and that there is reasonable assurance that it will not recur.

"(3) In lieu of the sanction authorized by paragraph (1), the Secretary may require that (as a condition to the continued eligibility of such practitioner or provider to provide such health care services on a reimbursable basis) such practitioner or provider pay to the United States, in case such acts or conduct involved the provision or ordering by such practitioner or provider of health care services which were medically improper or unnecessary, an amount not in excess of the actual or estimated cost of the medically improper or unnecessary services so provided, or (if less) $5,000. Such amount may be deducted from any sums owing by the United States (or any instrumentality thereof) to the person from whom such amount is claimed.

"(4) Any person furnishing services described in paragraph (1) who is dissatisfied with a determination made by the Secretary under this subsection shall be entitled to reasonable notice and opportunity for a hearing thereon by the Secretary to the same extent as is provided in section 205(b), and to judicial review of the Secretary's final decision after such hearing as is provided in section 205(g).

53 Stat. 1368.
42 USC 405.

"(c) It shall be the duty of each Professional Standards Review Organization and each Statewide Professional Standards Review Council to use such authority or influence it may possess as a professional organization, and to enlist the support of any other professional or governmental organization having influence or authority over health care practitioners and any other person (including a hospital or other health care facility, organization, or agency) providing health care services in the area served by such review organization, in assuring that each practitioner or provider (referred to in subsection (a)) providing health care services in such area shall comply with all obligations imposed on him under subsection (a).

"NOTICE TO PRACTITIONER OR PROVIDER

"SEC. 1161. Whenever any Professional Standards Review Organization takes any action or makes any determination—
"(a) which denies any request, by a health care practitioner or other provider of health care services, for approval of a health care service or item proposed to be ordered or provided by such practitioner or provider; or
"(b) that any such practitioner or provider has violated any obligation imposed on such practitioner or provider under section 1160,
such organization shall, immediately after taking such action or making such determination, give notice to such practitioner or provider of such determination and the basis therefor, and shall provide him with appropriate opportunity for discussion and review of the matter.

"STATEWIDE PROFESSIONAL STANDARDS REVIEW COUNCILS; ADVISORY GROUPS TO SUCH COUNCILS

Establishment.

"SEC. 1162. (a) In any State in which there are located three or more Professional Standards Review Organizations, the Secretary shall establish a Statewide Professional Standards Review Council.

Membership.

"(b) The membership of any such Council for any State shall be appointed by the Secretary and shall consist of—
"(1) one representative from and designated by each Professional Standards Review Organization in the State;
"(2) four physicians, two of whom may be designated by the State medical society and two of whom may be designated by the State hospital association of such State to serve as members on such Council; and
"(3) four persons knowledgeable in health care from such State whom the Secretary shall have selected as representatives of the public in such State (at least two of whom shall have been recommended for membership on the Council by the Governor of such State).

Duties.

"(c) It shall be the duty and function of the Statewide Professional Standards Review Council for any State, in accordance with regulations of the Secretary, (1) to coordinate the activities of, and disseminate information and data among the various Professional Standards Review Organizations within such State including assisting the Secre-

October 30, 1972   Pub. Law 92-603   <u>86 STAT. 1441</u>

tary in development of uniform data gathering procedures and operating procedures applicable to the several areas in a State (including, where appropriate, common data processing operations serving several or all areas) to assure efficient operation and objective evaluation of comparative performance of the several areas and, (2) to assist the Secretary in evaluating the performance of each Professional Standards Review Organization, and (3) where the Secretary finds it necessary to replace a Professional Standards Review Organization, to assist him in developing and arranging for a qualified replacement Professional Standards Review Organization.

"(d) The Secretary is authorized to enter into an agreement with Payments. any such Council under which the Secretary shall make payments to such Council equal to the amount of expenses reasonably and necessarily incurred, as determined by the Secretary, by such Council in carrying out the duties and functions provided in this section.

"(e)(1) The Statewide Professional Standards Review Council for any State (or in a State which does not have such Council, the Professional Standards Review Organizations in such State which have agreements with the Secretary) shall be advised and assisted in carrying out its functions by an advisory group (of not less than seven nor more than eleven members) which shall be made up of representatives of health care practitioners (other than physicians) and hospitals and other health care facilities which provide within the State health care services for which payment (in whole or in part) may be made under any program established by or pursuant to this Act.

"(2) The Secretary shall by regulations provide the manner in Member selection, which members of such advisory group shall be selected by the State- regulations. wide Professional Standards Review Council (or Professional Standards Review Organizations in States without such Councils).

"(3) The expenses reasonably and necessarily incurred, as deter- Expenses. mined by the Secretary, by such group in carrying out it duties and functions under this subsection shall be considered to be expenses necessarily incurred by the Statewide Professional Standards Review Council served by such group.

"NATIONAL PROFESSIONAL STANDARDS REVIEW COUNCIL

"SEC. 1163. (a)(1) There shall be established a National Profes- Establishment; sional Standards Review Council (hereinafter in this section referred membership. to as the 'Council') which shall consist of eleven physicians, not otherwise in the employ of the United States, appointed by the Secretary without regard to the provisions of title 5, United States Code, govern- 5 USC 101 <u>et</u> ing appointments in the competitive service. <u>seq.</u>

"(2) Members of the Council shall be appointed for a term of three Term of member- years and shall be eligible for reappointment. ship.

"(3) The Secretary shall from time to time designate one of the members of the Council to serve as Chairman thereof.

"(b) Members of the Council shall consist of physicians of recog- Qualifications. nized standing and distinction in the appraisal of medical practice. A majority of such members shall be physicians who have been recommended by the Secretary to serve on the Council by national organizations recognized by the Secretary as representing practicing physicians. The membership of the Council shall include physicians who have been recommended for membership on the Council by consumer groups and other health care interests.

"(c) The Council is authorized to utilize, and the Secretary shall Consultants. make available, or arrange for, such technical and professional consultative assistance as may be required to carry out its functions, and the

Pub. Law 92-603   **October 30, 1972**

Secretary shall, in addition, make available to the Council such secretarial, clerical and other assistance and such pertinent data prepared by, for, or otherwise available to, the Department of Health, Education, and Welfare as the Council may require to carry out its functions.

Compensation.

"(d) Members of the Council, while serving on business of the Council, shall be entitled to receive compensation at a rate fixed by the Secretary (but not in excess of the daily rate paid under GS-18 of the General Schedule under section 5332 of title 5, United States

5 USC 5332 note.

Code), including traveltime; and while so serving away from their homes or regular places of business, they may be allowed travel expenses, including per diem in lieu of subsistence, as authorized by section 5703 of title 5, United States Code, for persons in Government service employed intermittently.

Duties.

"(e) It shall be the duty of the Council to—
  "(1) advise the Secretary in the administration of this part;
  "(2) provide for the development and distribution, among Statewide Professional Standards Review Councils and Professional Standards Review Organizations of information and data which will assist such review councils and organizations in carrying out their duties and functions;
  "(3) review the operations of Statewide Professional Standards Review Councils and Professional Standards Review Organizations with a view to determining the effectiveness and comparative performance of such review councils and organizations in carrying out the purposes of this part; and
  "(4) make or arrange for the making of studies and investigations with a view to developing and recommending to the Secretary and to the Congress measures designed more effectively to accomplish the purposes and objectives of this part.

Report to Secretary and Congress.

"(f) The National Professional Standards Review Council shall from time to time, but not less often than annually, submit to the Secretary and to the Congress a report on its activities and shall include in such report the findings of its studies and investigations together with any recommendations it may have with respect to the more effective accomplishment of the purposes and objectives of this part. Such report shall also contain comparative data indicating the results of review activities, conducted pursuant to this part, in each State and in each of the various areas thereof.

"APPLICATION OF THIS PART TO CERTAIN STATE PROGRAMS RECEIVING FEDERAL FINANCIAL ASSISTANCE

"SEC. 1164. (a) In addition to the requirements imposed by law as a condition of approval of a State plan approved under any title of this Act under which health care services are paid for in whole or part, with Federal funds, there is hereby imposed the requirement that provisions of this part shall apply to the operation of such plan or program.

"(b) The requirement imposed by subsection (a) with respect to such State plans approved under this Act shall apply—
  "(1) in the case of any such plan where legislative action by the State legislature is not necessary to meet such requirement, on and after January 1, 1974; and
  "(2) in the case of any such plan where legislative action by the State legislature is necessary to meet such requirement, whichever of the following is earlier—
    "(A) on and after July 1, 1974, or

"(B) on and after the first day of the calendar month which first commences more than ninety days after the close of the first regular session of the legislature of such State which begins after December 31, 1973.

"CORRELATION OF FUNCTIONS BETWEEN PROFESSIONAL STANDARDS REVIEW ORGANIZATIONS AND ADMINISTRATIVE INSTRUMENTALITIES

"SEC. 1165. The Secretary shall by regulations provide for such correlation of activities, such interchange of data and information, and such other cooperation consistent with economical, efficient, coordinated, and comprehensive implementation of this part (including, but not limited to, usage of existing mechanical and other data-gathering capacity) between and among—

"(a) (1) agencies and organizations which are parties to agreements entered into pursuant to section 1816, (2) carriers which 79 Stat. 297. are parties to contracts entered into pursuant to section 1842, 42 USC 1395h. and (3) any other public or private agency (other than a Profes- 42 USC 1395u. sional Standards Review Organization) having review or control functions, or proved relevant data-gathering procedures and experience, and

"(b) Professional Standards Review Organizations, as may be necessary or appropriate for the effective administration of title XVIII, or State plans approved under this Act. 42 USC 1395.

"PROHIBITION AGAINST DISCLOSURE OF INFORMATION

"SEC. 1166. (a) Any data or information acquired by any Professional Standards Review Organization, in the exercise of its duties and functions, shall be held in confidence and shall not be disclosed to any person except (1) to the extent that may be necessary to carry out the purposes of this part or (2) in such cases and under such circumstances as the Secretary shall by regulations provide to assure adequate protection of the rights and interests of patients, health care practitioners, or providers of health care.

"(b) It shall be unlawful for any person to disclose any such infor- Penalty. mation other than for such purposes, and any person violating the provisions of this section shall, upon conviction, be fined not more than $1,000, and imprisoned for not more than six months, or both, together with the costs of prosecution.

"LIMITATION ON LIABILITY FOR PERSONS PROVIDING INFORMATION, AND FOR MEMBERS AND EMPLOYEES OF PROFESSIONAL STANDARDS REVIEW ORGANIZATIONS, AND FOR HEALTH CARE PRACTITIONERS AND PROVIDERS

"SEC. 1167.- (a) Notwithstanding any other provision of law, no person providing information to any Professional Standards Review Organization shall be held, by reason of having provided such information, to have violated any criminal law, or to be civilly liable under any law, of the United States or of any State (or political subdivision thereof) unless—

"(1) such information is unrelated to the performance of the duties and functions of such Organization, or

"(2) such information is false and the person providing such information knew, or had reason to believe, that such information was false.

"(b) (1) No individual who, as a member or employee of any Professional Standards Review Organization or who furnishes profes-

86 STAT. 1444

Pub. Law 92-603   October 30, 1972

sional counsel or services to such organization, shall be held by reason
of the performance by him of any duty, function, or activity authorized
or required of Professional Standards Review Organizations under
this part, to have violated any criminal law, or to be civilly liable
under any law, of the United States or of any State (or political subdivision thereof) provided he has exercised due care.

"(2) The provisions of paragraph (1) shall not apply with respect
to any action taken by any individual if such individual, in taking
such action, was motivated by malice toward any person affected by
such action.

"(c) No doctor of medicine or osteopathy and no provider (including directors, trustees, employees, or officials thereof) of health care
services shall be civilly liable to any person under any law of the
United States or of any State (or political subdivision thereof) on
account of any action taken by him in compliance with or reliance
upon professionally developed norms of care and treatment applied
by a Professional Standards Review Organization (which has been

Ante, p. 1430.   designated in accordance with section 1152(b)(1)(A)) operating in
the area where such doctor of medicine or osteopathy or provider took
such action but only if—

"(1) he takes such action (in the case of a health care practitioner) in the exercise of his profession as a doctor of medicine
or osteopathy (or in the case of a provider of health care services)
in the exercise of his functions as a provider of health care services, and

"(2) he exercised due care in all professional conduct taken or
directed by him and reasonably related to, and resulting from
the actions taken in compliance with or reliance upon such professionally accepted norms of care and treatment.

"AUTHORIZATION FOR USE OF CERTAIN FUNDS TO ADMINISTER THE
PROVISIONS OF THIS PART

"SEC. 1168. Expenses incurred in the administration of this part
shall be payable from—

"(a) funds in the Federal Hospital Insurance Trust Fund;
"(b) funds in the Federal Supplementary Medical Insurance
Trust Fund; and
"(c) funds appropriated to carry out the health care provisions
of the several titles of this Act;

in such amounts from each of the sources of funds (referred to in subsections (a), (b), and (c)) as the Secretary shall deem to be fair and
equitable after taking into consideration the costs attributable to the
administration of this part with respect to each of such plans and
programs.

"TECHNICAL ASSISTANCE TO ORGANIZATIONS DESIRING TO BE DESIGNATED
AS PROFESSIONAL STANDARDS REVIEW ORGANIZATIONS

"SEC. 1169. The Secretary is authorized to provide all necessary
technical and other assistance (including the preparation of prototype
plans of organization and operation) to organizations described in section 1152(b)(1) which—

"(a) express a desire to be designated as a Professional Standards Review Organization; and
"(b) the Secretary determines have a potential for meeting the
requirements of a Professional Standards Review Organization

October 30, 1972   Pub. Law 92-603   86 STAT. 1445

to assist such organizations in developing a proper plan to be submitted to the Secretary and otherwise in preparing to meet the requirements of this part for designation as a Professional Standards Review Organization.

"EXEMPTIONS OF CHRISTIAN SCIENCE SANATORIUMS

"SEC. 1170. The provisions of this part shall not apply with respect to a Christian Science sanatorium operated, or listed and certified, by the First Church of Christ, Scientist, Boston, Massachusetts."

Appendix C

Cross-References to the PSRO Law

PL 92-603* §249F	SSA**	42 USC#	Stat. at Large##
	1151	1320c	86 Stat 1429
	1152	1320c-1	86 Stat 1430
	1153	1320c-2	86 Stat 1432
	1154	1320c-3	86 Stat 1432
	1155	1320c-4	86 Stat 1433
	1156	1320c-5	86 Stat 1435
	1157	1320c-6	86 Stat 1437
	1158	1320c-7	86 Stat 1437
	1159	1320c-8	86 Stat 1437
	1160	1320c-9	86 Stat 1438
	1161	1320c-10	86 Stat 1440
	1162	1320c-11	86 Stat 1440
	1163	1320c-12	86 Stat 1441
	1164	1320c-13	86 Stat 1442
	1165	1320c-14	86 Stat 1443
	1166	1320c-15	86 Stat 1443
	1167	1320c-16	86 Stat 1443
	1168	1320c-17	86 Stat 1444
	1169	1320c-18	86 Stat 1444
	1170	1320c-19	86 Stat 1445
PL 94–182 §105	1152(g)	1320c-1(g)	89 Stat 1052

* PL 92–603: "Social Security Amendments of 1972 (H.R. 1)"
** Social Security Act
# United States Code, Title 42
United States Statutes at Large, volumes 86 and 89

108(a)	1152(c)&(f)	1320c-1(c)&(f)	89 Stat 1053
108(b)	none	none	89 Stat 1053
112(c)	1168	1320c-17	89 Stat 1055

Simplified Index to PSRO Guidelines

---

* M. stands for the *PSRO Program Manual*
** T. stands for Transmittal Letter
*** PMIS is the standard abbreviation for the *PSRO Management Information Systems Manual*

Appendix E

List of Transmittal Letters and Effective Dates

Transmittal Number	Subject	Date
1	Introduction	August 2, 1974
2	Planning preparation	August 2
3	BQA/OPSR structure	August 3
4	Support Centers: Reporting	August 8
5	Travel requests	August 21
6	Tax status	September 3
7	Continuing Education	October 1
8	Subcontracting	September 30
9	Data: Baselines	October 18
10	Transition in status (planning to conditional)	November 5
11	Delegation	November 21
12	Administrative Directors	December 5
13	UR: Regulations	—
14	State Agencies	January 31, 1975
15	Delegation: Reconsideration	February 12
16	Data: Confidentiality	February 14
17	AMA model criteria	February 18
18	Support Centers: Role	—
19	Advisory Groups	May 13
20	Data: Processing	May 30
21	UR: Relationship to PSRO	June 20
22	UR: Relationship to PSRO	June 20
23	UR: Regulations delayed	July 2
24	State Agencies	August 11
25	Data: Deliverables	August 26

26	Data: Processing	September 12
27	Delegation: Financing	December 18
28	Data: Deliverables	January 9, 1976
29	Hearings and Appeals	February 21
30	UR: Physician Certifications	February 27
31	Contract Management	March 2
32	Data: Notice to patients	March 2
33	HSAs: Area Designation	April 5
34	Delegation: Reimbursement	April 9
35	Travel and Salary Amounts	April 9
36	Civil Rights Responsibilities	April 30
37	PSRO Review of Non-federally Reimbursed Peer Review	June 28
38	Title V Relationships	July 2
39	Data: Routing and Processing	August 11
40	Program Decentralization	October 6
41	Data: Revised Confidentiality Standards	October 6
42	Data: Revised Reporting Requirements	October 6
43	M.C.E. Study Policy	January 25, 1977
44	Non-physicians in Short-stay Peer Review	January 25
45	Data: Routing and Processing, Integrating with Existing Systems	February 1
46	Reimbursement for Delegated Hospitals	March 11

Glossary

Agency: 1. A relationship in which one person or group acts for or represents another. The agent derives authority from either an express or implied agreement arising from the actions of the parties involved. 2. A person or group within the executive branch of government, appointed by the executive and acting for him within the limits set by the legislature and the courts.

Agreement: In the government contract context, a legally binding understanding of specified conditions that both parties approve, but are not necessarily dictated by federal regulations.

Administrative Law: That body of law dealing with the powers and procedures of agencies. Within the administrative structure agencies exercise quasi-legislative and judicial powers. Agency secretaries are frequently granted the power under law to promulgate regulations to implement a particular bill. Within agency powers are decision-making authorities that involve formal hearing and appeal procedures which are of a binding nature and must be exhausted prior to appeal in a judicial forum.

Administrative Procedures Act: A federal law passed in 1946 that establishes rulemaking and adjudicatory procedures for federal agencies.

Confidentiality: The protection of a communication made between two or more individuals.

Contributory Negligence: Action by an injured plaintiff that, combined with the negligent conduct of the defendant, was a cause of the plaintiff's injury.

Comparative Negligence: A method of apportioning liability according to negligence or fault. Under this method, if the fault of the plaintiff is equal or greater than the fault of the defendant, the plaintiff would not be entitled to recover.

Corporate Liability: A corporation as a separate legal entity is responsible for obeying the corporate laws of its respective state, its articles of incorporation and bylaws; failure to do so, if it results in injury, may render the corporation legally liable. A corporation is also legally responsible for the negligent acts or omissions of its employees and officers when they are acting on behalf of the corporation.

Defamation: The communication to third parties or party of false information which is injurious to the reputation of the individual referred to in the communication. Defamation can be either written (libel) or oral (slander).

Discovery: The procedures by which a litigant can compel disclosure by another party to the lawsuit of facts, deeds, documents or other things which are in that person's exclusive knowledge or possession and which are needed by the litigant as part of a specific cause of action.

Government Contract: A legally binding understanding executed between the government or one of its agents and another party, the terms and operation of which are controlled by federal regulations.

Malice: The intentional doing of a wrongful act without just cause or excuse, with an intent to inflict an injury or under circumstances from which the law will infer an evil intent.

Memorandum of Understanding: An agreement between two or more parties, often dealing with the provision of services, which sets down basic principles of cooperation between involved parties. Memoranda are often used at initial stages of negotiation and frequently lead to more formalized contracts.

Malpractice: Medical malpractice is a form of professional negligence in which measurable injury occurs to a plaintiff patient as the direct result of an act or omission by the defendant practitioner.

Privacy: The right of an individual person to keep information about him- or herself inaccessible.

Regulation: A rule, having the force of law, issued by an agency pursuant to a legislative mandate. Regulations promulgated by federal agencies must be developed according to the dictates of the Administrative Procedures Act.

Respondeat Superior: The principle that holds an employer responsible for the wrongdoings of his employees provided they are acting within the scope of their employment.

Rule-making: The process of issuing regulations under the Administrative Procedures Act, which involves a series of steps (varying with the agency), including notice of intent to publish regulations, public comment, issuance of proposed regulations, additional public comment, and finally, issuance of final regulations. Regulations are published in their various stages in the *Federal Register.*

Selected Bibliography

Chapter 1

Adamson, T. E. and Barbaccia, J. C. *A Curriculum for Teaching Medical Audit and Utilization Review.* San Francisco: University of California, 1974.

American Hospital Association. *Quality Assurance Program for Medical Care in the Hospital.* Chicago: American Hospital Association, 1972.

American Medical Association Council on Health Manpower. "Continuing Competence of Physicians." *Journal of American Medical Association* 217 (1971).

AMA Division of Medical Practice. *Peer Review, A Selection of Papers.* Chicago: American Medical Association, 1970.

American Medical Association. *Peer Review Manual,* Volumes I & II. Chicago: American Medical Association, 1971.

American Psychiatric Association. "Position on Peer Review in Psychiatry." *American Journal of Psychiatry* 130 (1973): 3.

Blue Cross of Massachusetts. *Pamphlet on Utilization Review Program.* Boston: Blue Cross of Massachusetts, 1975.

Brian, Earl. "Government Control of Hospital Utilization." *New England Journal of Medicine* 286 (1972): 1340.

Brook, Robert, and Appel, Francis. "Quality of Care Assessment: Choosing a Method for Peer Review." *New England Journal of Medicine* 288 (1973): 1323.

Buck, Charles R., and White, Kerr L. "Peer Review: Impact of a System Based on Billing Claims." *New England Journal of Medicine* 291 (1975): 877.

Byrant, Alice; O'Donoghue, Patrick; and Toerber, Garry. *Current Perceptions by the Health Care Community of the Activities of Four Western Foundations for Medical Care.* Denver: Spectrum Research, 1975.

Byrant, Alice, and Updegraff, Gail. *Regulations of Institutional Quality.* Denver: Spectrum Research, 1975.

California Medical Association. *Guidelines for Patient Care Evaluation.* San Francisco: California Regional Medical Program, 1975.

Colcock, Bentley P. "PSRO-Editorial." *New England Journal of Medicine* 290 (1974): 1318.

Decker, Barry, and Bonner, Paul. *PSRO Organization for Regional Peer Review.* Cambridge: Ballinger Publishing, 1973.

Donabedian, Avedis. "Promoting Quality through Evaluating the Process of Patient Care." *Medical Care* 6 (1968): 181.

Egdahl, Richard H. "Foundations for Medical Care." *New England Journal of Medicine* 288(1973): 491.

Flashner, Bruce; Reed, Shirley; White, Roger; and Norris, John. "The Hospital Admission and Surveillance Program in Illinois." *Journal of the American Medical Association* 221 (1972): 1153.

Foundation for Health Care Evaluation. *Technical Proposal to Health Services Administration for Operation as a Conditionally Designated PSRO in Minnesota PSRO Area II.* Minneapolis: Foundation for Health Care Evaluation, 1974.

Fox, Leslie; Stearns, Gerry; and Thompson, Richard. *PEP Workbook for Physicians and Committee Assistants.* Chicago: Joint Commission on Accreditation of Hospitals, 1975.

Frederick, Larry. "PSROs: How Are the First Ones Working." *Medical World News* 15 N.38 (1974):53

Gertman, Paul M. and Egdahl, Richard H., eds. *Quality Assurance in Health Care.* Germantown, Maryland: Aspen Systems Corporation, 1976.

Goldberg, George, and Holloway, Don. "Emphasizing Level of Care over Length of Stay in Hospital Utilization Review." *Medical Care* 13 (1975): 474.

Goldstein, Richard; Roberts, James *et seq.* "Data for Peer Review: Acquisition and Use." *Annals of Internal Medicine* 82 (1975): 262.

Goodman, Raymond, ed. *The Proceedings from PSRO, an Educational Symposium.* Los Angeles: University of California Department of Continuing Education in Health Sciences, 1975.

Gosfield, Alice. *PSROs: The Law and the Health Consumer.* Cambridge: Ballinger Publishing, 1975.

Harrington, Donald. "The San Joaquin Foundation Peer Review System." *Medical Care* 11 (1973): 185.

Joint Commission on Accreditation of Hospitals. *TAP Institutes.* Chicago: Joint Commission on Accreditation of Hospitals, 1972.

Lembeke, Paul. "Evolution of Medical Audit" *Journal of the American Medical Association* 199 (1967): 111.

Arthur D. Little. "Evolution of the Hawaii EMCRO." Cambridge: Arthur D. Little, 1974.

McCain, John. "The Background and Development of Peer Review." *Journal of the Medical Association of Georgia* 62 (1973): 336.

McKillop, William. "Quality of Care Evaluation: A Medical Process in a Public Domain." *Hospital Medical Staff* (1975): 10.

Mississippi PSRO. *Formal Plan for the Implementation of a Conditional PSRO.* Jackson: Mississippi PSRO, 1974.

Multnomah Foundation for Medical Care. *A Proposal for Operation as a Conditionally Designated PSRO.* Portland: Multnomah FMC, 1974.

New Mexico PSRO. *A Proposal to Be Designated a Conditional PSRO.* Albuquerque: New Mexico PSRO, 1974.

Payne, Beverly, ed. *Hospital Utilization Review Manual.* Ann Arbor: University of Michigan Medical School, 1968.

Pearce, H.G. "The Role of the Fiscal Intermediary in PSRO." *Hospital Medical Staff* 4 (1975): 30.

Richardson, Fred. "Peer Review of Medical Care." *Medical Care* 10 (1972): 29.

Sanazaro, Paul; Goldstein, Richard *et seq.* "Research and Development in Quality Assurance." *New England Journal of Medicine* 287 (1972): 1125.

Schlicke, Carl. "American Surgery's Noblest Experiment." *Arch Surg.* 106 (1973): 379.

Slater, Carl and Bryant, Alice. *Regulations of Professional Performance. Denver: Spectrum Research, 1975.*

Slee, Virgil. "PSRO and the Hospital's Quality Control." *Annals of Internal Medicine* 81 (1974): 97.

Tribble, William, and Ho, Yaw Chin. *A PSRO Health Care Review System.* Memphis: Tennessee Foundation for Medical Care, 1974.

Utah Professional Review Organization. *Quality Care Guidelines.* Salt Lake City: UPRO, 1974.

Utah Professional Review Organization. *UPRO Nurses Coordinator Handbook.* Salt Lake City: UPRO, 1974.

Waldman, Martin. "The Medical Audit Study—A Tool for Quality Control." *Hospital Progress* 54 Feb. (1973): 82.

Welch, Claude. "PSROs: Pros and Cons." *New England Journal of Medicine* 290 (1974): 1319.

Williamson, John; Alexander, Marshall; and Miller, George. "Priorities in Patient-Care Research and Continuing Medical Education." *Journal of the American Medical Association* 204 (1968).

Chapters 2, 3, and 4

Decker, Barry, and Bonner, Paul. *PSRO: Organization for Regional Peer Review.* Cambridge: Ballinger Publishing, 1973.

Egdahl, Richard H., Gertman, Paul M., et. al. *Quality Assurance in Hospitals: Policy Alternatives.* New York: Springer-Verlag New York, Inc., 1976.

Forgotsen, Cook. "Innovations and Experiments in the Use of Health Manpower—the Effect of Licensure Laws." *Law and Contemporary Problems* 32 (1967): 561.

Frederick, Larry. "PSROs: What Doctors Nationally Think of Them." *Medical World News* (October 25, 1974): 70.

Gauntt, William M. "Marketing Tax-Exempt Hospital Bonds: The Mechanics and Problems" in *Tax-Exempt Financing of Hospitals and Health Care Facilities.* New York: Practising Law Institute, 1975.

Jessee, William F., Munier, William B., et. al., "PSRO: An Educational Force for Improving Quality of Care." *New England Journal of Medicine* 292 (March 27, 1975): 668.

LeMaitre, George D. "PSROs and the Violation of Privacy." *PSRO Update,* No. 5 (September 1974): 2.

Mackey, Barbara. "Results of PSRO Balloting." *PSRO Update,* No. 25 (October 1976): 1.

Miller, Michael H. "PSROs—Boon or Bust for Nursing." *Hospitals* 49 (October 1, 1975): 81.

Reich, Charles. "The New Property." *Yale Law Journal* 73 (1964): 733.

Segal, Marshall B., "A Hard Look at the PSRO Law," *The Journal of Legal Medicine* 2 (September/October 1974): 16.

Snydert, James, and Robert Engelman. "PSROs—Time to Review the Peer Reviewers." *Modern Medicine* 45 (February 1, 1977): 52.

Spivak, Jonathan. "Medical-Care Review Stirs a Fiery Debate Among U.S. Doctors." *Wall Street Journal* (June 24, 1971): col. 1, p. 1.

Welch, Calude E. "PSROs—Pros and Cons." *New England Journal of Medicine* 290 (June 6, 1974): 1319.

Willett, David E. "PSRO Today: A Lawyer's Assessment." *New England Journal of Medicine* 292 (February 13, 1975): 340.

―――"Level of PSRO Funding Brings Question About the Intent of Congress," *PSRO Update*, No. 9 (June 3, 1975): 6.

―――*PSRO Program Manual.* Washington, D.C.: GPO, 197 .

―――*PSRO Management Information Systems Manual.* Washington, D.C.: GPO, 19 .

Chapter 5

Adams, A. "The National Railroad Passenger Corporation—A Modern Hybrid Corporation Neither Public Nor Private." *Business Law* 31 (1976) 601.

Davidson, J. F. *Administrative Law & the Regulatory Process.* Washington: Lerner Law Books, 1968.

Freedman, James. "Administrative Procedure & the Control of Foreign Direct Investment." *U. Pa. Law Review* 119 (1970): 6–9.

Jaffe, L. and Nathanson, N. *Administrative Law: Cases and Materials.* Boston: Little, Brown, 1968.

Orleans v. United States, 509 F.2d 197 (1975).

U.S. House of Representatives. *Conference Committee Report on the Freedom of Information Act.* H.R.93-1380, 1974.

Chapter 6

Andersen, Crystal, et al. "Privacy Invasion: Fighting Back the Threat." *Patient Care* January (1975): 107.

Bigelow, Robert. "The Privacy Act of 1974." *Practical Lawyer* 21 (1975): 17.

Clark, E. "Holding Government Accountable: The Amended Freedom of Information Act." *Yale Law Journal* 84 (1975): 741.

Boyer, Barry. "Computerized Medical Records and the Right to Privacy: The Emerging Federal Response." *Buffalo Law Review* 25 (1975): 37.

Curren; Laska; *et seq.* "Protection of Privacy and Confidentiality." *Science* 23 (1973): 197.

DHEW. *Records, Computers and the Rights of Citizens.* Washington: DHEW Publication Nos. 73–97, 1973.

———. *Instructions and Guidelines for Implementation of the DHEW Professional Standards Review Organization Confidentiality Policy.* Washington: Bureau of Quality Assurance, Health Services Administration, 1976.

———. *Transmittal Letter No. 16, Specifications for Confidentiality Policy on PSRO Data and Information.* Washington: Bureau of Quality Assurance, Health Services Administration, 1975.

Freed, Roy. "A Legal Structure for a National Medical Data Center." *Boston University Law Review* 49 (1969): 79.

Freedman, Alfred. "Looking over the Doctor's Shoulder." *Trial Magazine.* 11 No. 1 (1975): 28.

Harvard Center for Community Health & Medical Care. *PSRO Information and Consumer Choice: The Case for Public Disclosure of Health Services Data.* Boston: Harvard University, 1975.

Hullet, David. "Confidentiality of Statistical and Research Data and the Privacy Act of 1974." *Statistical Reporter* (June) 1975.

Lavett, William. "Private Actions for Deceptive Trade Practices." *Administrative Law Review* 23 (19): 271.

Miller, Arthur. "A Nation of Datamaniaes." *Prism* 2 (1974): 19.

New Mexico Foundation for Medical Care. *New Mexico PSRO Position Paper on Confidentiality.* Alburquerque: New Mexico PSRO, 1974.

Norris, John. "Legal Aspects of Computer Use in Patient Therapy." Boston: Paper delivered at the First National Conference on the Legal Aspects of Computer Use in Health Care Delivery, Nov. 7, 8, 1974.

Note. "The Freedom of Information Act: A Seven-year Assessment." *Columbia Law Review* 74 (1974): 895.

Note. "Freedom of Information Act: The Expansion of Exemption Six." *University of Florida Law Review* 28 (1975): 848.

Note. "The Freedom of Information Act: The Parameters of the Exception." *Georgetown Law Journal* 62 (1973): 177.

Note. "Right to Privacy: Social Interest and Legal Right." *Minnesota Law Review* 51 (1967): 531.

Note. "Roe and Paris, Does Privacy Have a Principle?" *Stanford Law Review* 26 (1974): 1161.

Renshaw, Charles. "Is Privacy Obsolete—The Challenge to Medicine and Society." *Prism* 2 (1974): 13.

Springer, Eric. "PSRO: A Perspective on Legal Liability and Confidentiality." PSRO Educational Symposium Monograph, UCLA Extension, Continuing Ed. in Health Sciences, 1975.

————. "Professional Standard Review Organizations: Some Problems of Confidentiality." *Utah Law Review* 1975 (Summer): 361.

Weed, Lawrence. "The Public's Need Must Be Met." *Prism* 2 (1974): 22.

Westin, Alan. *Privacy and Freedom.* New York: Atheneum Press, 1967.

U.S. House Republican Research Committee. *Recommendations of Privacy Task Force.* Washington: House Republican Research Committee, 1974.

Thomas, Richard. "The Medical Practice Computer Profile: Proof of the Doctor's Actions in a Series of Similar Cases." *University of California at Davis Law Review* 7 (1974): 523.

U.S. Senate Finance Committee. *Senate Finance Committee on H.R.1, Social Security Amendments of 1972.* Washington: Senate Finance Committee H.R. 92-1230.

Chapter 7

American Law Institute. *Restatement of the Law of Torts 2nd.* "Physicians and Surgeons" 19—.

Boikess, Olga and Winsten, Jay. "Can PSRO Procedures Be Both Fair and Workable." *Catholic University Law Review* 24 (1975): 407.

Curran, William and Shapiro, E. Donald. *Law, Medicine and Forensic Science.* Boston: Little, Brown, 1970.

DHEW. *Report of the Secretary's Commission on Medical Malpractice.* Washington: DHEW Publication Nos. 73–83, 1973.

Donoghue, Robin. "Admissibility of Medical Books in Evidence." *University of San Francisco Law Review* 8 (1973): 364.

Holder, Angela. *Medical Malpractice Law.* New York: John Wiley & Sons Inc., 1975.

Kramer, Charles. *Medical Malpractice.* New York: Practicing Law Institute, 1965.

McCormack, Charles T. *Evidence.* St. Paul: West Publishing, 1954.

Note. "Compliance with Professional Standards, Not Necessarily Absolving Factor." *Texas Tech Law Review* 6 (1974): 279.

Note. "PSRO and Medical Malpractice Liability." *Boston University Law Review* 54 (1974): 931.

Note. "PSRO: Malpractice Liability and the Impact of the Civil Immunity Clause." *Georgetown Law Review* 62 (1974): 1499.

Note. "Res Ipsa Loquitur: Its Place in Medical Malpractice Litigation." *University of San Francisco Law Review* 8 (19): 343.

Note. "Sources of a Physicians' Standard of Care." *Brigham Young University Law Review* (1975): 572.

Oleck, Howard. "New Medicolegal Standards of Skill and Care." *Cleveland-Marshall Law Review* 11 (1962): 443.

Springer, Eric. "PSRO: A Perspective on Legal Liability and Confidentiality." UCLA Extension PSRO Symposium Monograph, Jan. 1975: 60.

Chapter 8

American Law Institute. *Restatement of the Law of Agency 2d.* St. Paul: West, 1958.

———. *Restatement of Torts 2d.* St. Paul: West, 1939.

Blum, John. "Due Process in Hospital Peer Review." *New England Journal of Medicine* 291 (1976): 29

Health Law Center. *Problems in Hospital Law.* Germantown, Md.: Aspen Systems Corporation, 1974.

JCAH. *Guidelines for the Formulation of Medical Staff By-Laws, Rules and Regulations.* Chicago: JCAH, 1971.

Kauper, P. *Constitutional Law.* Boston: Little, Brown, 1972.

Prosser, D. *Law of Torts.* St. Paul: West, 1958.

Southwick, Arthur. "The Hospital as an Institution, Expanding Responsibilities Change Relationship with the Staff Physician." *Cal. Western Law Review* 9 (1973): 429.

Table of Cases

A

B

C

*The letter "n" indicates that the case is discussed in a footnote.

D

F

G

H

T

U

V

W

Y

Z

Index

About the Authors

John D. Blum is presently a member of the Boston University Health Policy Center where he is engaged in teaching and research activities in the health law field. Mr. Blum is a contributing editor to PSRO Update and is a lecturer in health policy in the B.U. Political Science Department. Prior to joining the Health Policy Center, Mr. Blum was a research associate in the Health Care Research Section of Boston University Medical School during which time he was a lecturer on the legal aspects of the PSRO program for a number of HEW training programs. Mr. Blum's principal areas of interest are health law, administrative law and public health policy. Blum is a graduate of Canisius College, Notre Dame Law School and the Harvard School of Public Health.

Paul M. Gertman, chief of the Health Care Research Section, Boston University School of Medicine (BUSM), also serves as director of the Health Service Research and Development Program of Boston University Medical Center and director of the Quality Assurance Unit of University Hospital, Boston. He is an assistant professor of medicine and surgery at BUSM. Among Dr. Gertman's principal current research interests are the economic costs to society of various approaches to cancer management, the tradeoffs between preventive and primary-care medicine, and the concept of preventable hospital admissions. He received his A.B. and M.D. degrees from Johns Hopkins University and was a Carnegie-Commonwealth Clinical Scholar there. While on duty with the U.S. Public Health Service, Dr. Gertman was research director of the President's Advisory Council on Management Improvement, a staff member of the Office of Science and Technology, and special assistant to the director of the National Center for Health Services Research and Development.

Jean Rabinow, now residing in New York City, was formerly special counsel to University Hospital in Boston and a member of the Health Care Research Section at Boston University Medical School. Ms. Rabinow's chief area of interest is hospital law, a field in which she has written and lectured extensively. Rabinow is a graduate of Knox College and the Yale Law School.